Life Saving Skills Manual

Essential Obstetric and Newborn Care

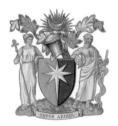

Royal College of
Obstetricians and
Gynaecologists

Setting standards to improve women's health

IN PARTNERSHIP WITH

**LIVERPOOL
SCHOOL OF
TROPICAL
MEDICINE**

**World Health
Organization**

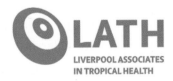
LATH
LIVERPOOL ASSOCIATES
IN TROPICAL HEALTH

Published by the **RCOG Press** at the Royal College of Obstetricians and Gynaecologists, 27 Sussex Place, Regent's Park, London NW1 4RG

www.rcog.org.uk

Registered charity no. 213280

First published 2006, revised 2007

ISBN 978-1-904752-28-8

Author: Nynke van den Broek DTM+H, FRCOG, PhD

RCOG Editor: Jane Moody
Design/typesetting by Karl Harrington, FiSH Books
Index by Liza Furnival
Printed by Bell & Bain, 303 Burnfield Road, Thornliebank, Glasgow G46 7UQ

Contents

Acknowledgements

The following people very kindly gave freely of their time to review this manual and made valuable suggestions for improvements.

Many thanks to: Kate Grady, consultant anaesthetist; Edwin Djabatey, consultant anaesthetist; John Williams, Sanjeev Sharma, Matthews Mathai, Alison Kirkpatrick and Peter Jackson, consultant obstetricians and gynaecologists; and the students of the 2006 Diploma in Reproductive Health course, especially Charles Ameh and Joanna Arnold.

Thank you most sincerely to the World Health Organization for permission to use the very clear pictures and diagrams from their publication: *Integrated Management of Pregnancy and Childbirth*.

Finally, thank you to Jane Moody at the RCOG for her unflinching support through the publication process.

Nynke van den Broek
June 2007

Introduction

Each year, more than 529 000 women worldwide die from complications of pregnancy and childbirth – that is one every minute. Many more survive but will suffer ill health and disability as a result of these complications. At least 80% of deaths result from five complications that are well understood and can be readily treated: haemorrhage, sepsis, eclampsia, obstructed labour and complications of abortion (Figure 1). We know how to prevent these deaths – there are existing effective medical and surgical interventions that are relatively inexpensive. The health of the neonate is closely related to that of the mother and an estimated 70% of deaths in the first month of life could also be prevented if interventions were in place to ensure good maternal health.

The reduction of maternal and neonatal mortality is one of the key goals of the Millennium Declaration. An important part of reaching this goal is the provision of **skilled attendance** and **essential (or emergency) obstetric care (EOC)** for pregnant women during labour, delivery and the immediate postpartum period.

Pregnancy should be a normal life event for the majority of women and yet every pregnancy faces risk. There is nothing as normal as a normal pregnancy and nothing as abnormal as an abnormal one – and nothing can go so quickly from one to the other. For an estimated 15% of all women, this complication will be unexpected and life threatening unless she has access to essential (or emergency) obstetric care. Having the skills to recognise and then respond effectively to such unexpected events is a key part of a skilled attendant's role.

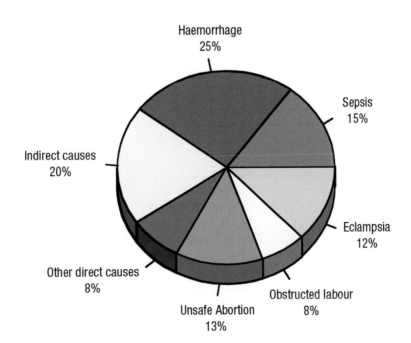

The term 'skilled attendant' refers to someone who has been educated and trained to proficiency in the skills needed to manage normal pregnancies, childbirth and the immediate postnatal period, and in the identification, management and referral of complications in women and newborns.

Basic emergency obstetric care (BEOC) consists of six key functions:

■ intravenous or intramuscular antibiotics
■ intravenous or intramuscular oxytocic drugs
■ intravenous or intramuscular anticonvulsants
■ manual removal of placenta
■ removal of retained products of conception
■ assisted vaginal delivery.

Comprehensive emergency obstetric care (CEOC) consists of all of the above functions plus the ability to provide:

■ caesarean section
■ blood transfusion.

This manual is structured around the leading causes of maternal mortality and the delivery of basic and comprehensive emergency obstetric care. It is meant for use by all those healthcare providers who mainly work in resource-poor settings, trying to save lives in sometimes very difficult situations. These include midwives, clinical officers, medical assistants and doctors. We sincerely applaud them and hope they will find this manual useful.

Nynke van den Broek
Jim Dornan
Monir Islam

Module 1
Communication, triage and referral

Aim

- To practise effective communication skills in emergency situations.
- To practise effective triage, emergency management and referral in obstetric emergencies.
- To achieve competency in the skills required.

Communication

All care should be based on the following standards:

Humanity	Women treated with respect
Benefit	Care based on the best available evidence
Commitment	Health professionals committed to improving care

Privacy and confidentiality

In all contacts with the woman and her partner:

- Ensure a private place for the examination and counselling.
- Ensure, when discussing sensitive subjects, that you cannot be overheard.
- Make sure that you have the woman's consent before discussing with her family.
- Never discuss confidential information about clients outside the health facility.
- Organise the examination area so that, during examination, the woman is protected from the view of other people (curtain, screen, wall).
- Ensure all records are confidential and kept locked away.

Triage and referral

'Triage' means to 'sift as through a sieve' or in other words **to prioritise.**

This term is used to mean:

1. **A quick assessment of an individual woman and her baby (born or unborn)**

and (in order to)

2. **Prioritise the order of treatment and allocation of staff e.g. in a labour ward with more than one patient.**

Both scenarios will now be described:

1. A quick assessment of an individual woman and her baby (born or unborn)

A person responsible for initial reception of women (pregnant or postpartum) and baby seeking care should:

■ assess the general condition immediately on arrival (if a woman is very sick, talk to her companion).

Ask, Check, Record
■ Why did you come?
   ☐ for yourself?
   ☐ for the baby?
■ How old is the baby?
■ What is the concern?

Look, Listen, Feel

Woman:
■ bleeding vaginally
■ convulsing
■ looking very ill
■ unconscious
■ in severe pain
■ in labour
■ delivery is imminent.

Baby:
■ very small
■ convulsing
■ breathing with difficulty.

Classify as one of the following:

Emergency for woman	Labour	Emergency for baby	Routine care

Emergency for woman

If the woman is:
■ unconscious
■ convulsing
■ bleeding from the vagina

If the woman has:
■ severe abdominal pain
■ headache and visual disturbance
■ severe difficulty breathing
■ high fever
■ severe vomiting

If the woman looks very ill

Treat
■ Transfer woman to a treatment room for RAPID assessment and management.
■ Call for help.
■ Reassure the woman that she will be taken care of immediately.
■ Ask her companion to stay.

Labour

- Frequent uterine contractions
- Rupture of membranes
- Imminent delivery

Treat

- Transfer the woman to the labour ward
- Call for immediate assessment

Emergency for baby

If the baby is:
- very small
- just born

If he has:
- convulsions
- difficult breathing

If there is any maternal concern

Treat

- Transfer the baby to the treatment room for immediate newborn care.
- Ask the mother to stay with the baby if she can.

Routine care

- Pregnant woman, or after delivery, with no danger signs
- A newborn with no danger signs

Treat

- Keep the woman and baby in the waiting room for routine care.
- If the woman is pregnant (and not in labour), provide antenatal care.
- If the woman has recently given birth, provide postpartum care.

2. Prioritise the order of treatment and allocation of staff

(For example, in a labour ward with more than one patient.)

The aim is to do the 'most for the most' and do this in the right order.

There are generally three categories of patients:

Priority 1:   **A woman who requires emergency treatment and resuscitation soon or she may die**
(for example, a woman in hypovolaemic shock or a woman with convulsions).

Priority 2:   **A woman whose care may be delayed for a few hours**
(for example, a woman with rupture of membranes – no prolapsed cord).

Priority 3:   **A woman who can sustain a significant delay**
(for example, a woman with a breech presentation who is not in labour).

[!]   The management of care in the labour ward is a dynamic process and regular reassessment of priorities is vital.

Referral

The **right** patient has to be taken at the **right** time by the **right** people to the **right** place using the **right** form of transport and receiving the **right** type of care throughout.

A good transfer is well planned and prepared.

This can be done by following the **ACCEPT** approach:

A: Assessment

Assess the situation. Sometimes the person who has given care to the woman until now will also accompany her on the transfer but often it is someone else who takes over the care during transfer. They will not have any prior knowledge of the woman's condition.

C: Control

Take control: identify who is in charge, identify what needs to be done and who is going to do it. Allocate tasks if possible.

Make sure the woman is accompanied by:

- a health worker trained in delivery care
- relatives who can donate blood
- baby with the mother
- essential emergency drugs and supplies for transfer
- referral note.

C: Communication

It is very important that the woman and her relatives are aware and informed of what is happening.

Transfer of a patient also requires the cooperation and involvement of several healthcare providers. Identify the key people involved and inform them as well and as early as possible.

Pass on information clearly and unambiguously (verbally and on paper if possible).

Important information to pass on is:

- who you are
- what are the patient's relevant details
- what is the problem
- what has been done so far to address the problem
- what is needed.

E: Evaluation

The risks of transfer must be balanced against the risks of staying and the benefit of care that can only be given by the receiving centre. For example, a critically ill woman may need transfer because she needs:

- basic obstetric care and is in the village
- needs comprehensive obstetric care and is in a BEOC facility.

Once it has been established that transfer is needed, it is also important to evaluate the urgency. The degree of urgency for transfer and the severity of the woman's condition will help to decide the mode of transport and the type of person to accompany her.

P: Preparation and packaging

Preparation involves ensuring that the woman's condition is as stable as possible and that it is safe to transport her.

The aim is to ensure that there is no change in the level of care provided during transfer and that there is no further deterioration in the woman's condition during transfer.

Ensure that adequate resuscitation has been carried out (for example, the airway clear, IV line in place).

All equipment must be functioning.

Supplies of drugs and fluids should be more than adequate for the whole of the journey.

All IV lines, catheter (if applicable) should be secured to the patient.

The patient should be secured in her position during the transfer.

All written documents (such as case notes, antenatal records, handover letter) should accompany the patient.

T: Transportation

The standard of care received before transfer needs to be maintained as much as possible during transport.

Monitoring of the woman's condition should continue during the transfer.

During the journey:

- watch IV infusion
- if journey is long, give appropriate treatment on the way
- keep a record of all IV fluids, medications given, time of administration and the woman's condition.

At the end of the transfer, direct contact must be made with the receiving person who will take over care of the woman. All documents should be handed over and a full explanation given of the course of events up to now.

Example of emergency drugs that may be needed during transfer

Emergency drugs	Emergency supplies
Oxytocin	Gloves
Ergometrine	Set for giving IV fluids
Magnesium sulphate	IV fluids
Diazepam (parenteral)	Sterile syringes and needles
Calcium gluconate	Urinary catheter
Ampicillin	Antiseptic solution
Gentamicin	Container for sharps
Metronidazole	Bag for rubbish
Ringer lactate	Torch and extra battery

If delivery is anticipated on the way:
Soap, towels
Disposable delivery kit (blade, 3 ties)
Clean cloths (3) for receiving, drying and wrapping the baby
Plastic bag for placenta
Resuscitation bag and mask for the baby

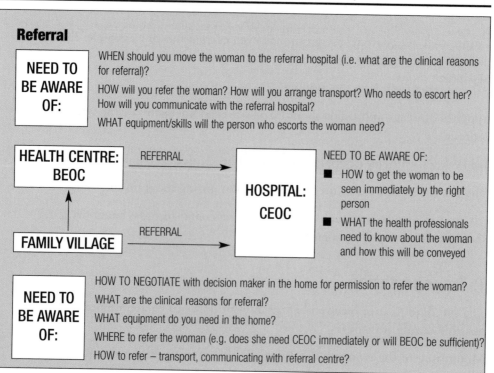

Referral

NEED TO BE AWARE OF:

WHEN should you move the woman to the referral hospital (i.e. what are the clinical reasons for referral)?

HOW will you refer the woman? How will you arrange transport? Who needs to escort her? How will you communicate with the referral hospital?

WHAT equipment/skills will the person who escorts the woman need?

HEALTH CENTRE: BEOC → REFERRAL → **HOSPITAL: CEOC**

FAMILY VILLAGE → REFERRAL →

NEED TO BE AWARE OF:
- HOW to get the woman to be seen immediately by the right person
- WHAT the health professionals need to know about the woman and how this will be conveyed

NEED TO BE AWARE OF:

HOW TO NEGOTIATE with decision maker in the home for permission to refer the woman?

WHAT are the clinical reasons for referral?

WHAT equipment do you need in the home?

WHERE to refer the woman (e.g. does she need CEOC immediately or will BEOC be sufficient)?

HOW to refer – transport, communicating with referral centre?

Module 2
Resuscitation of mother and neonate

Aim

■ To understand and be able to practise resuscitation of the mother and the neonate.

Resuscitation of the mother

The approach to an apparently lifeless patient is the cardiopulmonary resuscitation (**ABC**) drill:

■ a rapid assessment of Airway and Breathing and correction of problems as they are found, moving through to correction of the absence of Circulation.

Adult resuscitation

■ Ensure a safe environment for patient and rescuer.
■ Shake and shout and, if no response, call for help and return to patient.

If patient appears lifeless:

■ Turn patient on to her back and place wedge under right side of abdomen to relieve aortocaval compression.

■ **Open the airway:**
   ☐ Remove any obvious obstruction from mouth.
   ☐ Perform head tilt by placing hand on patient's forehead and tilting the head back.
   ☐ Perform chin lift by placing two fingers under the point of the patient's chin and lifting the chin forward.
   ☐ Jaw thrust, performed by placing fingers behind patient's jaw and lifting jaw forward, may be necessary.

■ **Assess breathing for 10 seconds:**
   ☐ Look for chest movements.
   ☐ Listen for breath sounds.
   ☐ Feel for movement of air.

If there is absence of breathing in the presence of an open airway, take this as an absence of circulation.

- If the patient is breathing, turn her in to the recovery position.
- If the patient is not breathing, give 30 chest compressions followed by two breaths.
  - ☐ Chest compressions are delivered to the middle of the lower half of the sternum.
  - ☐ Place the heel of your first hand on top of the patient, put the other hand on top and interlock the fingers of both hands. Keep in midline to ensure that pressure is not applied over the ribs. Do not apply pressure over the abdomen or bottom tip of the sternum.
  - ☐ Lean well over the woman and, with your arms straight, press down vertically on the sternum to depress it approximately 4–5 cm at a rate of 100 compressions/ minute. Change the person delivering the compressions every two minutes but avoid delays in changeover.

Breaths are delivered by taking a full breath and placing your lips around the mouth and blowing steadily into the mouth. If possible, a facemask and self-inflating bag or pocket mask should be used. Maintain head tilt and chin lift when giving breaths. Each breath should last about one second and should make the chest rise as with a normal breath.

If available, oxygen should be given as soon as possible.

If CPR unsuccessful after 4–5 minutes, perform caesarean section. This is urgent to reduce the pressure of the pregnant uterus on the maternal vessels. The patient does not need to be moved to the operating theatre.

- Consider and treat causes of cadiopulmonary arrest:
  - ☐ **Four Hs:**
    Hypoxia
    Hypovolaemia
    Hyperkalaemia and other metabolic disorders
    Hypothermia (very unlikely)
  - ☐ **Four Ts:**
    Thromboembolism (pulmonary embolism or amniotic fluid embolism)
    Toxicity
    Tension pneumothorax (very unlikely)
    Cardiac tamponade (very unlikely)

Resuscitation and care of the newborn

General principles:

- Hands should be washed and gloves worn before touching the newborn.
- Tell the woman (and her support person) what is going to be done, listen to her and respond attentively to her questions and concerns.
- Provide continual emotional support and reassurance, as feasible.

Assessment table

Initial assessment	Action
Pink	
Breathing regularly	Dry and wrap
Heart rate more than 100 beats/minute	Give baby to the mother
Blue	
Breathing inadequately	Dry and wrap
Heart rate 60 beats/minute or less	Open airway
	Inflation breaths
Blue or white	
Not breathing	Dry and wrap
Heart rate less than 60 beats/minute	Open airway
	Inflation breaths
	Reassess
	Do you need help?

Start resuscitation within 1 minute of birth if the baby is not breathing or is gasping for breath. Initially, an assessment of heart rate is made, by listening with a stethoscope at the apex of the heart. This is done because heart rate is used to assess the effectiveness or otherwise of the resuscitation process to follow. Once the baby has a patent airway it is very likely to resuscitate spontaneously.

■ Call for help.
■ Start the clock.
■ Dry the baby, wrap in a fresh towel and keep warm.
■ Assess initially by listening with a stethoscope at the apex.

Note: the heart rate is a guide to the success of resuscitation.

The Apgar score is then calculated at 1 and 5 minutes and is a tool for evaluating baby's condition at birth. It is not used to guide resuscitation. It assesses:

■ BREATHING — rate and quality (airway and breathing)
■ HEART RATE — fast, slow, absent (circulation)
■ COLOUR — pink, blue, pale (circulation)
■ TONE — unconscious, apnoeic babies are floppy (airway, breathing and circulation).

The Apgar scoring system

System	Score		
	0	1	2
Heart rate	Absent	Below 100/minute	100/minute or higher
Respiratory effort	Nil	Slow, irregular	Regular, with cry
Muscle tone	Limp	Some tone in limbs	Active flexion of limbs
Reflex irritability	Nil	Grimace only	Cry
Colour	Pallor or generalised cyanosis	Body pink, extremities blue	Pink all over

Airway:

- Position the head in the neutral position to open the airway. Overextension or flexion will collapse the pharyngeal airway. A towel folded to 2–3 cm thickness placed under the shoulders will help to achieve the correct position.
- Most babies, even those born not breathing, will resuscitate themselves given a clear airway.
- If the baby is floppy, use the jaw thrust to bring the tongue forward and open the airway.
- Very gentle suction of the oropharynx or nostril **ONLY** using a soft suction catheter may be used. Deep suction is dangerous and should not be used – it can cause bradycardia and spasm of the larynx.
- In the unconscious baby, airway obstruction is usually due to loss of pharyngeal muscle tone and to foreign material in the airway. Simply opening the airway will solve the problem.

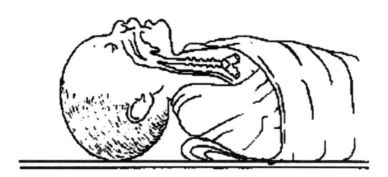

Breathing:

If the baby does not respond to opening the airway as described above:

- Place the mask (attached to the bag) firmly over the newborn's mouth, chin and nose, to form a seal between the mask and the newborn's face.
- Using bag and mask, give five inflation breaths, each of 2–3 seconds.
- Check the rise of the chest. The chest may not move during the first one to three inflation breaths, which are needed to displace fluid from the lungs.
- Check the seal and that the chest rises and falls with inflation breaths after that.
- Reassess the heart rate after the first five breaths: an increasing heart rate or a heart rate maintained at more than 100 beats/minute is a sign of adequate ventilation. If the heart rate has not responded check again for chest movement and check for patent airway when attempting to deliver ventilations.
- Ventilation should be continued at 30–40 breaths/minute.

Circulation:

If there is no heartbeat or the heartbeat is less than 60 beats/minute, even when the chest is being ventilated, give chest compressions. However, the most common reason for the heart rate remaining low is that successful ventilation has not been achieved.

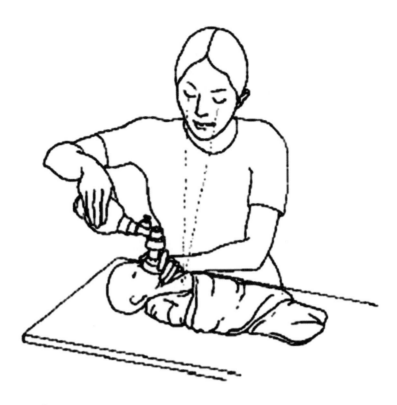

Chest compressions:

■ The best way to give cardiac massage is to encircle the baby's chest with two hands so that the thumbs meet on the sternum below the line between the nipples (see below). Compress chest by one-third of its depth – three times for each inflation.

■ Once the heart rate is above 60/minute and rising, chest compressions can be discontinued.

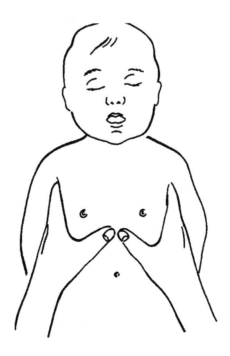

If the baby's breathing is normal (30–60 breaths/minute) and there is no indrawing of the chest and no grunting:

■ Put in skin-to-skin contact with mother.

■ Observe breathing at frequent intervals.

■ Measure the newborn's temperature and re-warm if temperature is less than 36°C.

■ Keep in skin-to-skin contact with mother.

■ Encourage mother to begin breastfeeding.

■ Keep the baby under observation until she or he has been stable for at least 6 hours.

■ Explain what happened to the mother.

If there is no gasping or breathing at all after 20 minutes of ventilation, or gasping but no breathing after 30 minutes of ventilation, stop ventilating.

Provide emotional support to the family.

DO NOT IN ANY CASE:

■ slap, blow on, or pour cold water on the baby

■ hold the baby upside down

■ routinely suction the mouth and nose of a well baby

■ use heavy suctioning of the back of the throat of any baby

■ give injections of respiratory stimulants or routine sodium bicarbonate injections.

Module 3
Shock and the unconscious patient

Aim

- To recognise shock.
- To practise the response to a woman in shock related to an obstetric emergency.
- To learn to grade levels of unconsciousness.
- To practise the response to an unconscious woman related to an obstetric emergency.

Shock

The focus in this module will be on the two main causes of shock and maternal death:

- haemorrhage
- sepsis.

Shock is a life-threatening condition that requires immediate and intensive treatment.

Shock means there is inadequate perfusion of organs and cells with oxygenated blood.

Recognising shock

Main signs and symptoms	Other signs and symptoms
Pulse weak and fast (> 110 beats/minute)	Pallor
BP low (systolic < 90 mmHg) (late sign)	Sweatiness or cold and clammy skin
	Rapid breathing
	Anxious, confused
	Unconscious
	Fetal distress

Action

1. Call for help.

2. Position the woman on her left side with her legs higher than her chest. Remember – in the pregnant woman any shock is made worse by aorta–caval compression.

3. Insert at least one IV line:
    ○ give fluids at rapid rate (see below)
    ○ if not able to insert peripheral IV lines, consider a cut-down (see below).

4. Keep her warm (cover her).

5. Assess the condition of mother and child.

The two most common causes of shock are haemorrhage and sepsis.

■ Bleeding vaginally or history of bleeding vaginally, follow management as for haemorrhage (Module 5).
■ If no bleeding and suspected sepsis – follow management as for sepsis (Module 7).

At health centre level (or BEOC):

6. Once initial treatment has commenced refer her urgently to hospital (CEOC).

Reassessment and further management

1. Reassess the woman's response to IV fluids within 30 minutes for signs of improvement:
    ○ stabilising pulse (90 beats/minute or less)
    ○ increasing systolic blood pressure (100 mmHg or more)
    ○ improving mental status (less confusion or anxiety)
    ○ increasing urine output (30 ml/hour or more).

2. If the woman's condition improves:
    ○ adjust the rate of IV infusion to 1 litre in 6 hours
    ○ continue management of underlying cause of shock.

Fluid management

1. Insert IV line and give fluids:
    ○ clean woman's skin with spirit at site for IV line
    ○ insert an IV line using a 16–18 gauge needle
    ○ attach Ringer lactate or normal saline

2. Give fluids at rapid rate if shock, systolic blood pressure (BP) less than 90 mmHg, pulse faster than 110 beats/minute or heavy vaginal bleeding:
    ○ infuse 1 litre in 15–20 minutes (as rapid as possible)
    ○ after that, infuse 1 litre in 30 minutes at 30 ml/minute
    ○ repeat if necessary.

3. Monitor every 15 minutes for:
    ○ pulse and BP
    ○ shortness of breath or puffiness.

4. Reduce the infusion rate:
    ○ to 3 ml/minute (1 litre in 6–8 hours) when pulse slows to less than 100 beats/minute, systolic BP increases to 100 mmHg or higher.
    ○ to 0.5 ml/minute if breathing difficulty or puffiness develops.

5. Give fluids at:
    ○ **moderate rate** if severe abdominal pain, obstructed labour, ectopic pregnancy, dangerous fever or dehydration: infuse 1 litre in 2–3 hours.
    ○ **slow rate** if severe anaemia/severe pre-eclampsia or eclampsia: infuse 1 litre in 6–8 hours.

6. Monitor urine output – insert a urinary catheter if available.

7. Record time and amount of fluids given – always use a **fluid balance sheet**.

Note: If IV access is not possible:
    ○ give oral rehydration solution (ORS) by mouth if able to drink, or by nasogastric (NG) tube, 300–500 ml in 1 hour.
    DO NOT give ORS to a woman who is unconscious or has convulsions.
    ○ Consider performing a venous cut-down to obtain IV access.

Procedure for venous cut-down

[!]   the saphenous vein is about one finger anterior and superior to the medial malleolus (on inner side ankle).

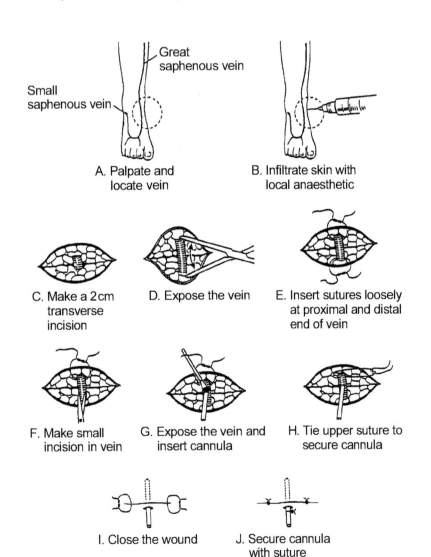

A. Palpate and locate vein

B. Infiltrate skin with local anaesthetic

C. Make a 2 cm transverse incision

D. Expose the vein

E. Insert sutures loosely at proximal and distal end of vein

F. Make small incision in vein

G. Expose the vein and insert cannula

H. Tie upper suture to secure cannula

I. Close the wound

J. Secure cannula with suture

Classification of circulating volume lost

[!] a pregnant woman has a circulation volume of about 100 ml/kg (for a woman of 60 kg this is 6 litres).

Class	Circulating volume lost	Signs
1	15% or less (not much more than 700 ml)	You may notice only a mild rise in pulse rate If the woman is otherwise healthy and if not anaemic she will not require a blood transfusion
2	15–30% (over 1.5 litres)	Symptoms will include rising pulse rate and rising breathing frequency Use crystalloids to replace fluid loss
3	30–40% (over 2 litres)	It is only at this stage that the blood pressure falls Remember a drop in BP is a late sign of hypovolaemia Patient will need a blood transfusion in addition to crystalloids
4	>40%	This is immediately life threatening Blood transfusion is required immediately

Patients with a reduced level of consciousness

- A rapid assessment of conscious level is made using **A V P U**:
- Is the patient **Alert**, responding to **Voice** or only responding to **Pain** or **Unresponsive**.

A decrease in the level of consciousness is the marker of insult to the brain (lack of oxygen). The more deeply the patient is (or becomes) unconscious, the more serious the insult.

Lack of oxygen to the brain results from either reduced blood flow (such as hypovolaemia) or reduced oxygen (caused, for example, by reduced breathing, convulsions, sepsis, anaemia).

- Call for help.
- Position woman on her left side.
- Assess Airway and Breathing (**Module 2**).

Not breathing

If the woman is not breathing or her breathing is shallow:

- Check airway.
- If she is not breathing, assist ventilation using Ambu-bag and mask or Laerdel pocket mask (Module 2).

    [!]   a patient with a reduced level of consciousness is likely to have an airway problem, as the tongue falls back into the throat and may be swollen because of tongue bite after convulsions.

- Assess circulation.
- Insert IV access (Circulation).
- Assess pregnancy state (pregnant or delivered).
- Assess **A V P U**
- Assess cause of reduced level of consciousness:
  - ☐ has there been a recent convulsion (eclampsia)?
  - ☐ is she a known epileptic?
  - ☐ is there any neck stiffness (meningitis)?
  - ☐ does she have a fever (temperature > 38°C)?
- Assess pupils (to check if cerebral bleed has occurred).
- Carry out observations of vital signs: pulse, breathing, blood pressure, temperature, fetal heart.

Convulsions

Eclampsia is the most common cause of unconsciousness. Remember, eclampsia can occur before, during or after delivery.

If the woman has had a convulsion or is convulsing: give magnesium sulphate (see **Module 4**).

High BP

If diastolic BP greater than 110 mmHg: give antihypertensive (see **Module 4**).

Fever

If temperature greater than 38 degrees C or history of fever, consider:

- sepsis
- malaria
- meningitis
- pneumonia.

Treat accordingly.

Always start specific therapy for condition leading to shock as soon as possible!

Module 4
Severe pre-eclampsia and eclampsia

Aim

- To recognise severe pre-eclampsia and eclampsia.
- To practise an effective response to a woman with severe pre-eclampsia or eclampsia.
- To achieve competency in the skills required.

Recognising severe pre-eclampsia

- BP greater than 140/90
- Proteinuria 2+ or more
- Headache
- Blurred vision
- Epigastric pain, upper abdominal pain
- Hyperreflexia, clonus
- Jittery
- Breathlessness (pulmonary oedema)
- Reduced urine output (less than 25 ml/hour or less than 100 ml/4 hours)

Principles of management

The cure for pre-eclampsia (and eclampsia) is delivery of the fetus and placenta. However, a rushed delivery in an unstable patient is incorrect. Only if severe hypertension and hypoxia in the mother have been corrected can delivery be expedited.

Treat hypertension if systolic BP is 170 mmHg or over, or diastolic BP is 110 mmHg or over. Aim to reduce BP to 130–140/90–100 mmHg. Commonly used antihypertensive drugs are hydralazine, labetalol and nifedipine.

Give steroids to promote lung maturity in a fetus of gestational age of less than 37 weeks.

Consider the need for magnesium sulphate:
- magnesium sulphate is given if eclampsia seems imminent and/or there is significant hyperreflexia and clonus (more than 3 beats) on clinical examination (severe pre-eclampsia).
- magnesium sulphate is given in all cases of eclampsia (fitting/convulsions).

Mode of delivery is decided at senior level after vaginal examination to assess the possibility of induction of labour.

Eclampsia

Recognising eclampsia

Convulsing (now or recently): tonic–clonic spasms like epilepsy

OR

Unconscious: if unconscious, ask relative "Has there been a recent convulsion?"

[!] A small proportion of women with eclampsia have a normal blood pressure. Treat all women with convulsions as if this is eclampsia until another diagnosis is confirmed.

Action
■ Do not leave the woman on her own: call for help.
■ Place woman into the left lateral position.
■ Maintain airway at all times.
■ Insert IV cannula and give fluids slowly (normal saline or Ringer lactate).
■ 1 litre in 6–8 hours (3 ml/minute or 30 drops per minute).
■ **Start magnesium sulphate.**

Magnesium sulphate
■ Magnesium sulphate ($MgSO_4$) is given as a **loading dose** followed by a **maintenance dose.**
■ The maintenance dose is continued for 24 hours after the delivery or after the last convulsion.
■ Magnesium sulphate can be given intramuscularly or intravenously (see the regimens below).

Intravenous regimen

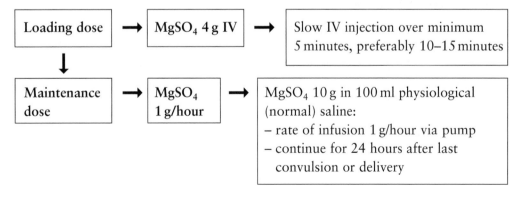

Intramuscular regimen

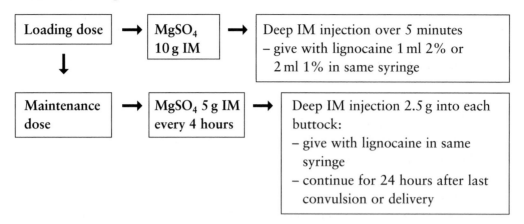

Note: If possible, give at least loading dose intravenously:

e.g. MgSO$_4$ 4 g IV loading then MgSO$_4$ % g 4-hourly IM

For IV maintenance dose a pump is needed.

DO NOT give the next dose of magnesium sulphate if any of these signs:

- knee jerk absent
- urine output less than 100 ml/4 hours
- respiratory rate less than 16 breaths/minute.

[!] Rapid injection may cause respiratory failure or death.

- If respiratory depression (breathing less than 16 breaths/minute) occurs after magnesium sulphate, do not give any more magnesium sulphate. Give the antidote: calcium gluconate 1 g IV (10 ml 10% solution) over 10 minutes.

If convulsions recur:

- After 15 minutes, give an additional 2 g of magnesium sulphate (10 ml of 20% solution) IV over 20 minutes. If convulsions still continue, give diazepam.

After receiving magnesium sulphate a woman may feel flushing, thirst, headache, nausea or may vomit.

[!] DO NOT give intravenous fluids rapidly (1 litre in 6–8 hours, or 3 ml/minute or 30 drops/minute).

[!] DO NOT give 50% magnesium sulphate intravenously without diluting it to 20%.

Management of high blood pressure

[!] A small proportion of women with eclampsia have a normal blood pressure. Treat all women with convulsions as if this was eclampsia until another diagnosis is confirmed.

If diastolic BP is greater than 110 mmHg or systolic BP 170 mmHg or above, give antihypertensive.

GIVE APPROPRIATE ANTIHYPERTENSIVE DRUG:

[!] Neither magnesium sulphate nor diazepam is antihypertensive: give hydralazine or labetalol or nifedipine.

- **Hydralazine** 5 mg IV slowly (3–4 minutes). If IV not possible, give IM.
  - ☐ If diastolic BP remains above 90 mmHg, repeat the dose at 30-minute intervals until diastolic BP is around 90 mmHg.
  - ☐ DO NOT give more than 20 mg in total.
  - ☐ If hydralazine is not available, give labetalol or nifedipine.
- **Labetalol** 10 mg IV.
  - ☐ If response is inadequate (diastolic BP remains above 110 mmHg) after 10 minutes, give labetalol 20 mg IV.
  - ☐ Increase dose to 40 mg and then 80 mg if satisfactory response is not obtained after 10 minutes of each dose.
- **Nifedipine** 5 mg orally.
  - ☐ If response to nifedipine is inadequate (diastolic remains above 110 mmHg) after 10 minutes, give an additional 5 mg.

Other points of management

1. **Monitor urine output:**
   - using a catheter if possible
   - check for proteinuria 4-hourly
   - keep a fluid input and output chart.

[!] DO NOT give intravenous fluids rapidly (30 drops/minute).

2. **Measure temperature:**
   - If temperature higher than 38 degrees C or history of fever, also give treatment for fever (antimalarials and/or antibiotics).

3. **Assess pregnancy status:**
   - If a woman with eclampsia is pregnant:
     - ○ delivery should take place as soon as the woman's condition has stabilised
     - ○ delivery should occur regardless of the gestational age.

4. **Assess the cervix:**
   - If the cervix is favourable (soft, thin, partly dilated), rupture the membranes and induce labour using oxytocin.
   - If the cervix is unfavourable (firm, thick, closed) ripen the cervix using misoprostol, prostaglandins or a Foley catheter.
   - If the baby is premature (gestational age is thought to be less than 37 completed weeks) and delivery is not imminent, give corticosteroids to reduce risk of respiratory distress syndrome and perinatal death.
   - Consider delivery by emergency caesarean section:
     - ○ if vaginal delivery is not anticipated within 12 hours
     - ○ if the cervix is unfavourable
     - ○ if there are fetal heart abnormalities (less than 100 beats/minute or more than 180 beats/minute).
   - If safe anaesthesia is not available for caesarean section or if the fetus is dead or too premature for survival, aim for vaginal delivery.

Diazepam

[!] **Magnesium sulphate is the drug of first choice in all circumstances and should be easily available at both BEOC and CEOC levels.**

Give diazepam:

■ if convulsions occur in early pregnancy

OR

■ if magnesium sulphate toxicity occurs

OR

■ If magnesium sulphate is not available.

Giving diazepam IV

■ Loading dose IV: give diazepam 10 mg IV slowly over 2 minutes.
■ If convulsions recur, repeat 10 mg.

Diazepam: vial containing 10 mg in 2 ml

Dose	Administration	
	IV	Rectally
Initial	10 mg = 2 ml	20 mg = 4 ml
Second	10 mg = 2 ml	10 mg = 2 ml

Diazepam maintenance dose:

■ Give diazepam 40 mg in 500 ml IV fluids (normal saline or Ringer lactate) titrated over 6–8 hours to keep the woman sedated but able to be roused.
■ Stop the maintenance dose if breathing rate less than 16 breaths/minute.
■ Assist ventilation if necessary with mask and bag.
■ Do not give more than 100 mg in 24 hours.
■ If IV access is not possible (e.g. during convulsion), give diazepam rectally.

Giving diazepam rectally:

■ Loading dose: give 20 mg (4 ml) in a 10 ml syringe (or urinary catheter).
■ Remove the needle, lubricate the barrel and insert the syringe into the rectum to half its length.
■ Discharge the contents and leave the syringe in place, holding the buttocks together for 10 minutes to prevent expulsion of the drug.
■ If convulsions recur, repeat 10 mg.
■ Maintenance dose: give additional 10 mg (2 ml) every hour during transport.

[!] The airway may need to be maintained and/or protected after diazepam treatment.

Module 5

Haemorrhage

Aim

■ To recognise an obstetric haemorrhage.
■ To practise the response to a woman with obstetric haemorrhage.

Risk of occurrence

BLEEDING can occur during:

Early pregnancy	Abortion (see **Module 10**)
	Ectopic pregnancy
Pregnancy	Placental abruption
	Placenta praevia
Labour	Placental abruption
	Placenta praevia
	Ruptured uterus
After delivery	Ruptured uterus
	Uterine atony
	Trauma (cervical, vaginal or labial tears)
	Retained placenta
	Retained products

ANY BLEEDING IS DANGEROUS BLEEDING

For management of all haemorrhage, always start with **A, B** then **C:**

A – secure **A**irway

B – **B**reathing

C – **C**irculation – commence IV and STOP bleeding.

General management

Assess bleeding by inspection:

[!] Do not conduct vaginal examination until placenta praevia has been excluded.

- Commence IV fluids immediately.
- Take blood for haemoglobin and crossmatching.
- Restore circulating volume; if the woman is in shock, follow **Management of Shock, Module 3.**

Then manage according to cause identified, as below.

General principles:

- Empty uterus; deliver fetus if not delivered.
- Remove placenta or retained products of conception.
- Give oxytocics (see below).
- Massage and bimanual compression of uterus.
- Compression of the aorta (temporary control).
- Repair of genital tract injury.
- Laparotomy with repair of rupture of uterus or subtotal hysterectomy.

Causes of bleeding in pregnancy

Presenting symptom and other symptoms and signs		Probable diagnosis
Usually present	**Sometimes present**	
Bleeding (vaginal or may be retained in the uterus = concealed) Intermittent or constant abdominal pain	Shock Tense, tender uterus Decreased/absent fetal movements Fetal distress or absent fetal heart sounds	Placental abruption
Bleeding (intra-abdominal and/or vaginal) Severe abdominal pain (may decrease after rupture)	Shock Abdominal distension/free fluid Abnormal uterine contour Tender abdomen Easily palpable fetal parts Absent fetal movements and fetal heart sounds Rapid maternal pulse	Ruptured uterus
Bleeding from the vagina	Shock Bleeding may be precipitated by intercourse Relaxed uterus Fetal presentation not in pelvis Normal fetal condition	Placenta praevia

Placental abruption

Placental abruption is the separation of the placenta from the uterus before the baby is delivered.

Blood collects in the space between the placenta and the uterus. It may leak out via the cervix (evident abruption) or accumulate behind the placenta (hidden or concealed abruption). In either case, blood loss is usually significant, the mother may be in hypovolaemic shock and there is lack of oxygen to the baby (poor or absent fetal heart rate).

The uterus is tender and hard (no relaxation between contractions). This is known as a 'woody', hard uterus or 'uterus en bois' or couvelaire uterus.

If bleeding is heavy (mother in shock or hypovolaemic or heavy bleeding from the vagina), deliver as soon as possible:

- If the cervix is fully dilated, deliver by vacuum extraction.
- If vaginal delivery is not imminent, deliver by caesarean section.

[!] in every case of placental abruption, be prepared for postpartum haemorrhage.

If bleeding is light to moderate (the mother is not in immediate danger), the course of action depends on the fetal heart rate.

- **If the fetal heart rate is normal or absent**, rupture the membranes.
- If contractions are poor, augment labour with oxytocin.
- If the cervix is unfavourable (firm, thick, closed), perform a caesarean section.
- **If the fetal heart rate is abnormal** (less than 100 or more than 180 beats/minute), perform vaginal delivery
- If vaginal delivery is not possible, deliver by immediate caesarean section.

Ruptured uterus

- Restore blood volume by infusing IV fluids (normal saline or Ringer lactate) before surgery.
- When stable, immediately perform laparotomy and deliver the baby and placenta (if not already delivered).
- If the uterus can be repaired with less operative risk than hysterectomy would entail and the edges of the tear are not necrotic, repair the uterus.
- If the uterus cannot be repaired, perform subtotal hysterectomy.
- If the tear extends through the cervix and vagina, total hysterectomy may be required (see **Module 6**).

Placenta praevia

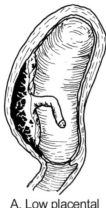 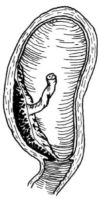 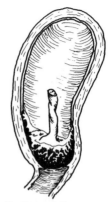

A. Low placental
   implantation

B. Partial placenta
   praevia

C. Complete
   placenta praevia

[!] **Do not perform vaginal examination unless preparations have been made for
immediate caesarean section.**

■ Restore blood volume by infusing IV fluids (normal saline or Ringer lactate).
■ Assess the amount of bleeding.
■ **If bleeding is heavy and continuous,** arrange for caesarean section delivery,
irrespective of fetal maturity or fetal condition.
■ **If bleeding is light or if it has stopped and the fetus is alive but premature,**
consider expectant management at centre offering CEOC until delivery or heavy
bleeding occurs:
    ☐ keep the woman in hospital until delivery
    ☐ correct anaemia (iron tablets, antimalarials, anthelminthics)
    ☐ ensure that blood is available for transfusion if required.
■ **If bleeding recurs,** decide management after weighing up benefits and risks for
the woman and fetus of further expectant management versus delivery.
■ If gestational age is less than 37 weeks, give corticosteroids for lung ripening.

Confirming diagnosis

■ If a reliable ultrasound examination can be performed to localise the placenta,
confirm the diagnosis of placenta praevia and if the fetus is mature (37 weeks of
gestation or more), plan delivery.
■ If ultrasound is not available and the pregnancy is less than 37 weeks, manage
as placenta praevia until 37 weeks.
■ If ultrasound is not available and the pregnancy is 37 weeks or more, examine
the woman in theatre and be prepared for either vaginal or caesarean section
delivery, as follows:
    ☐ have IV lines running and cross-matched blood available
    ☐ examine the woman in the operating theatre with the surgical and
       anaesthesia teams present
    ☐ use a sterile vaginal speculum to examine the cervix.
■ If the cervix is partly dilated and placental tissue is visible (placenta praevia is
confirmed), deliver by caesarean section.

■ If the cervix is not dilated, cautiously palpate the vaginal fornices:
  ☐ if spongy tissue is felt (placenta praevia is confirmed), deliver by caesarean section
  ☐ if a firm fetal head is felt (major placenta praevia is ruled out), proceed to deliver by induction of labour unless haemorrhage occurs.

Specific other problems to note

Bleeding with severe abdominal pain

This may be caused by, for example, ruptured uterus, obstructed labour, placental abruption, puerperal or post-abortion sepsis, ectopic pregnancy.

■ Severe abdominal pain (not normal labour).
■ Measure blood pressure (see Module 3).
■ Measure temperature.
■ If temperature more than 38 degrees C, start IM/IV antibiotics (see Module 7).

Clotting failure

Pregnancy complications in which coagulation failure is likely to occur are:

■ placental abruption
■ pre-eclampsia
■ eclampsia
■ sepsis
■ intrauterine death – retained dead fetus
■ amniotic fluid embolism.

Note: In cases of prolonged (massive) postpartum haemorrhage clotting failure can also occur.

In case of clotting failure, it is often necessary to use blood products to help control haemorrhage.

■ Give fresh whole blood, if available, to replace clotting factors and red cells.
■ If fresh whole blood is not available, choose one of the following based on availability:
  ☐ fresh frozen plasma for replacement of clotting factors (15 ml/kg body weight)
  ☐ cryoprecipitate to replace fibrinogen
  ☐ platelet concentrates.

Causes of vaginal bleeding after delivery

Presenting symptom and other symptoms and signs		Probable diagnosis
Usually present	**Sometimes present**	
Postpartum haemorrhage Uterus soft and not contracted	Shock	Atonic uterus
Postpartum haemorrhage Uterus contracted	Complete placenta	Episiotomy Tears of cervix, vagina or perineum
Postpartum haemorrhage	Placenta not delivered within 30 minutes after delivery	Retained placenta
Portion of maternal surface of placenta missing or torn membranes	Postpartum haemorrhage Uterus contracted	Retained placental fragments
Uterine fundus not felt on abdominal palpation	Inverted uterus apparent at the vulva	Inverted uterus
Pain Bleeding occurs more than 24 hours after delivery Uterus softer and larger than expected	Postpartum haemorrhage Bleeding is variable (light or heavy, continuous or irregular) and may be foul smelling Anaemia	Secondary postpartum haemorrhage
Postpartum haemorrhage (bleeding is intra-abdominal and/or vaginal) Severe abdominal pain	Shock Tender abdomen	Ruptured uterus

Postpartum haemorrhage

Recognising postpartum haemorrhage
- Bleeding with:
  - ☐ pad or cloth soaked in less than 5 minutes
  - ☐ constant trickling of blood
  - ☐ bleeding more than 500 ml

OR

- Delivered outside health centre and still bleeding.

Management
- Call for extra help.
- Massage uterus until it is hard and give oxytocin 10 units IM.
- Give IV fluids with 20 units oxytocin at 60 drops/minute.
- Empty bladder: catheterise if necessary.
- Check and record BP and pulse every 15 minutes.
- Establish the cause of bleeding.

Haemorrhage, placenta not delivered
- Check and ask if placenta is delivered.
- When uterus is hard, deliver placenta by controlled cord traction.
- If unsuccessful and bleeding continues, remove placenta manually and check placenta.
- Give appropriate IM/IV antibiotics.
- If unable to remove placenta, refer woman urgently to hospital.
- During transfer, continue IV fluids with 20 units oxytocin at 30 drops/minute.

Haemorrhage, placenta delivered
- Check placenta.
- If placenta is complete:
  - massage uterus to express any clots
  - if uterus remains soft, give ergometrine 0.2 mg IV
  - DO NOT give ergometrine to women with eclampsia, pre-eclampsia or known hypertension but give oxytocin instead
  - continue IV fluids with 20 units oxytocin/litre at 30 drops/minute
  - continue massaging uterus until it is hard.
- If placenta is incomplete (or not available for inspection):
  - remove placental fragments
  - give appropriate IM/IV antibiotics
  - if unable to remove, refer woman urgently to hospital.

Perineal and vaginal tears
- Examine the tear and determine the degree and extent of the tear.
- If third-degree tear (involving rectum or anus), refer woman urgently to facility with CEOC.
- For other tears: apply pressure over the tear with a sterile pad or gauze and put legs together. Do not cross ankles.
- Check after 5 minutes; if bleeding persists, repair the tear.

For repair of episiotomy and tears see **Module 8 Assisted delivery**.

Use of oxytocic drugs
Heavy bleeding:

- Check if still bleeding.
- Continue IV fluids with 20 units oxytocin at 30 drops/minute.
- Insert second IV line if necessary.

Controlled bleeding:

- Continue oxytocin infusion with 20 units/litre IV fluids at 20 drops/minute for 4–6 hours after bleeding stops.

Use of oxytocic drugs

Drug	Dose and route	Continuing dose	Maximum dose	Precautions and contraindications
Oxytocin	IV: infuse 20 units in 1 litre IV fluids at 60 drops/ minute IM: 10 units	IV: infuse 20 units in 1 litre IV fluids at 40 drops/minute	Not more than 3 litres IV fluids containing oxytocin	Do not give as an IV bolus
Ergometrine	IM or IV (slowly) L 0.2 mg	Repeat 0.2 mg IM after 15 minutes If required, give 0.2 mg IM or IV (slowly) every 4 hours	Five doses (total 1.0 mg)	High blood pressure Pre-eclampsia Heart disease
15-methyl prostaglandin F_2 (carboprost)	IM: 0.25 mg	0.25 mg every 15 minutes	Eight doses (total 2 mg)	Asthma

Manual removal of placenta

Preparation

1. Prepare the necessary equipment.

2. Tell the woman (and her support person) what is going to be done, listen to her and respond attentively to her questions and concerns.

3. Provide continual emotional support and reassurance, as feasible.

4. Have the woman empty her bladder or insert a catheter, if necessary.

5. Give anaesthesia (IV pethidine and diazepam or ketamine).

6. Give a single dose of prophylactic antibiotics:
   ○ ampicillin 2 g IV PLUS metronidazole 500 mg IV

      OR

   ○ cefazolin 1 g IV PLUS metronidazole 500 mg IV.

7. Put on personal protective equipment.

Procedure

1. Use antiseptic hand rub or wash hands and forearms thoroughly with soap and water and dry with a sterile cloth or air dry.

2. Put high-level disinfected or sterile surgical gloves on both hands.

   [!] Elbow-length gloves should be used, if available.

3. Hold the umbilical cord with a clamp.

4. Pull the cord gently until it is parallel to the floor.

5. Place the fingers of one hand into the vagina and into the uterine cavity, following the direction of the cord until the placenta is located.

6. When the placenta has been located, let go of the cord and move that hand on to the abdomen to support the fundus abdominally and to provide counter-traction to prevent uterine inversion.

7. Move the fingers of the hand in the uterus laterally until the edge of the placenta is located.

8. Keeping the fingers tightly together, ease the edge of the hand gently between the placenta and the uterine wall, with the palm facing the placenta.

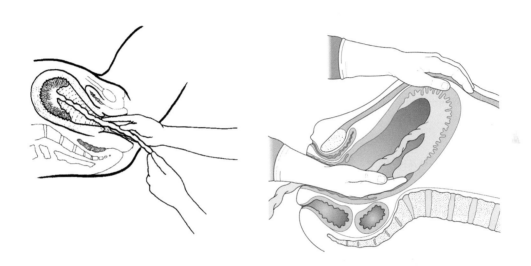

9. Gradually move the hand back and forth in a smooth lateral motion until the whole placenta is separated from the uterine wall.

    [!] If the placenta does not separate from the uterine wall by gentle lateral movement of the fingers at the line of cleavage, suspect placenta accrete and arrange for surgical intervention.

10. When the placenta is completely separated:
    ○ palpate the inside of the uterine cavity to ensure that all placental tissue has been removed
    ○ slowly withdraw the hand from the uterus, bringing the placenta with it
    ○ continue to provide counter-traction to the fundus by pushing it in the opposite direction of the hand that is being withdrawn.

11. Give oxytocin 20 units in 1 litre IV fluid (normal saline or Ringer lactate) at 60 drops/minute.

12. Have an assistant massage the fundus to encourage atonic uterine contraction.

13. If there is continued heavy bleeding, give ergometrine 0.2 mg IM or give prostaglandins (haemabate, carboprost; See Appendix 3).

14. Examine the uterine surface of the placenta to ensure that it is complete.

15. Examine the woman carefully and repair any tears to the cervix or vagina, or repair episiotomy.

Post-procedure

1. Immerse both gloved hands in 0.5% chlorine solution. Remove gloves by turning them inside out.

   [!] If disposing of gloves, place them in a leakproof container or plastic bag. If reusing surgical gloves, submerge them in 0.5% chlorine solution for 10 minutes for decontamination.

2. Use antiseptic hand rub or wash hands thoroughly with soap and water and dry with a clean, dry cloth or air dry.

3. Monitor vaginal bleeding and take the woman's vital signs:
   ○ every 15 minutes for 1 hour
   ○ then every 30 minutes for 2 hours.

4. Make sure that the uterus is firmly contracted.

5. Record procedure and findings on woman's record.

Inverted uterus

This is said to happen when the uterus turns inside out during delivery of the placenta.

Repositioning should be performed immediately as, with time elapsing, a constricting ring around the uterus becomes more rigid and the uterus more engorged with blood.

This may be accompanied by bleeding or sometimes is 'dry'.

- Commence IV fluids immediately as for general management of haemorrhage.
- Give pethidine IV/IM 1 mg/kg (not more than 100 mg) (or morphine 0.1 mg/kg IM).
- [!] DO NOT give any oxytocic drugs until inversion is corrected.
- If the placenta is still attached, do not attempt to remove this until after the uterus has been repositioned.
- Use one of the techniques below to reposition the uterus.

Repositioning of uterus

Manual repositioning

- If possible give anaesthesia (but all delay should be avoided).
- Under sterile conditions (if possible) reposition uterus by pushing uterus back.
- Push the whole mass first into the vagina then through the cervix and then finally into the normal position.

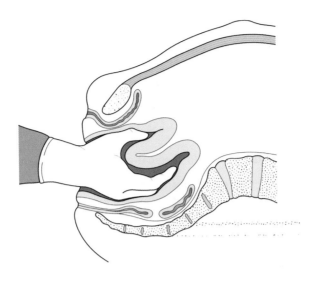

Hydrostatic repositioning

■ Exclude uterine rupture first.

■ Infuse warm saline into the vagina via a rubber tube held 1–2 metres above the patient while an assistant blocks the vaginal orifice.

■ It may be easier to do this by attaching the IV giving set to a silicone ventouse cup inserted into the vagina as this gives a better seal.

■ Drugs can be given to relax the cervical ring to facilitate replacement:
  □ magnesium sulphate 2–4 g given IV over 5 minutes.
  □ ritodrine 0.15 mg IV bolus.

Surgery

If above techniques do not work, it will be necessary to use surgery.

■ Perform a laparotomy and reposition the uterus either by:
  □ pulling from above using Allis' forceps placed in the dimple of the inverted uterus and gentle gradual upward traction (Huntington's procedure)

  OR

  □ cut the cervical ring posteriorly, using a longitudinal incision first (Haultain's technique).

After repositioning
■ If placenta not removed do so manually.
■ Ensure oxytocics given to keep uterus contracted.
■ Give antibiotics to prevent infection (if not already commenced).

Bimanual compression of the uterus

Preparation
1. Tell the woman (and her support person) what is going to be done, listen to her and respond attentively to her questions and concerns.

2.   Provide continual emotional support and reassurance, as feasible.

3.   Put on personal protective equipment.

Procedure

1.   Use antiseptic hand rub or wash hands thoroughly with soap and water and dry with a sterile cloth or air dry.

2.   Put high-level disinfected or sterile surgical gloves on both hands.

3.   Clean the vulva and perineum with antiseptic solution.

4.   Insert one hand into the vagina and form a fist.

5.   Place the fist into the anterior vaginal fornix and apply pressure against the anterior wall of the uterus.

6.   Place the other hand on the abdomen behind the uterus.

7.   Press the abdominal hand deeply into the abdomen and apply pressure against the posterior wall of the uterus.

8.   Maintain compression until bleeding is controlled and the uterus contracts.

Post-procedure

1.   Immerse both gloved hands in 0.5% chlorine solution. Remove gloves by turning them inside out.

   [!] When disposing of gloves, place them in a leakproof container or plastic bag.

2.   Use antiseptic hand rub or wash hands thoroughly with soap and water and dry with a clean, dry cloth or air dry.

3.   Monitor vaginal bleeding and take the woman's vital signs:
   ○ every 15 minutes for 1 hour
   ○ then every 30 minutes for 2 hours.

4.   Make sure that the uterus is firmly contracted.

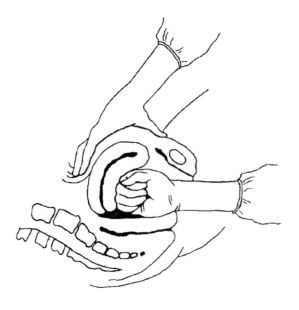

Compression of the abdominal aorta

Preparation

1. Tell the woman (and her support person) what is going to be done, listen to her and respond attentively to her questions and concerns.

2. Provide continual emotional support and reassurance, as feasible.

   [!] Steps 1 and 2 should be implemented at the same time as the following steps.

Procedure

1. Place a closed fist just above the umbilicus and slightly to the left.

2. Apply downward pressure over the abdominal aorta directly through the abdominal wall.

3. With the other hand, palpate the femoral pulse to check the adequacy of compression:
   ○ if the pulse is palpable during compression, the pressure is inadequate
   ○ if the pulse is not palpable during compression, the pressure is adequate.

4. Maintain compression until bleeding is controlled.

Post-procedure

1. Monitor vaginal bleeding and take the woman's vital signs:
   ○ every 15 minutes for 1 hour
   ○ then every 30 minutes for 2 hours.

2. Make sure that the uterus is firmly contracted.

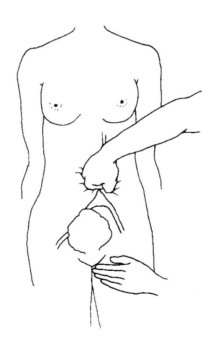

Module 6
Obstructed labour

Aim

- To recognise obstructed labour.
- To practise the skills needed to respond effectively to a woman who is in obstructed labour.
- To achieve competency in the skills required.

Appendix 1 contains a summary of supporting normal labour and use of the partograph and should be referred to during this module.

Labour is prolonged if a woman is in labour for more than 12 hours without delivery.

Partograph

- The partograph (or partogram) is a structured graphical representation of the progress of labour. It shows cervical dilatation in relation to time as well as descent of the fetal head. Space can be provided to write notes on, for example, frequency of contractions, fetal heart rate, maternal observations and medication given.
- Unsatisfactory progress in labour occurs when cervical dilatation is to the right of the alert line on the partograph.
- The partograph is simple to use and with its use the progress of labour can be seen at a glance on one sheet of paper. Failure to progress can be easily recognised.
- The partograph should be started once a woman is in labour.
- All women in labour should be monitored using a partograph.

Definitions

The following terms are used:

Latent phase   From the onset of labour up to a dilatation of 3–4 cm when the active phase begins.

Active phase   From this point (3–4 cm dilatation) there is usually progressive dilatation of the cervix at about 1cm/hour.

A partograph is started once a woman is diagnosed to be in labour; that is, with regular contractions (three in 10 minutes) each lasting 40 seconds or more. Failure to progress in labour may be because of problems with the:

Powers: Contractions inadequate.

Passage: Pelvis too small for baby.

Passenger: Position wrong or baby too large for pelvis.

[!] **It is very important to decide which of the three causes contribute to failure to progress so that appropriate action is taken.**

Dysfunctional labour is said to occur if contractions are inadequate.

Cephalopelvic disproportion occurs because the passenger (fetus) is too large or the passage (pelvis) is too small. If labour persists in the presence of cephalopelvic disproportion it may become arrested (contraction decrease or stop) or obstructed. Once cephalopelvic disproportion is confirmed, delivery is by caesarean section.

First stage of labour

Findings suggestive of unsatisfactory progress:

- irregular and infrequent contractions after the latent phase

   AND/OR

- cervical dilatation slower than 1cm/hour during the active phase of labour (cervical dilatation to the right of the alert line)

   AND/OR

- cervix poorly applied to the presenting part.

Management
- If uterine contractions are infrequent and/or irregular:
  - ☐ ensure use of partograph
  - ☐ encourage mobility and oral hydration
  - ☐ rupture the membranes with amniotic hook or a Kocher clamp
  - ☐ augment labour using oxytocin
  - ☐ reassess progress by vaginal examination 2 hours after a good contraction pattern with strong contractions has been established.
- If no progress between examinations, deliver by caesarean section.

Second stage of labour

Findings suggestive of unsatisfactory progress:

- lack of descent of fetus through birth canal
- failure of expulsion.

Management

- Allow spontaneous pushing.
- Encourage change of maternal position/mobility.
- If malpresentation and obvious obstruction have been excluded, and contractions are inadequate, consider whether to augment labour with oxytocin.

If no descent after augmentation:

- If the fetal head is not more than two-fifths palpable above the symphysis pubis or the fetal head is at the spines or lower, deliver by vacuum extraction (see **Module 8**).
- If the fetal head is more than two-fifths palpable above the symphysis pubis or the leading bony edge of the fetal head is above −2 station, deliver by caesarean section.
- If caesarean section is not possible and the operator is proficient in symphysiotomy, this may also be considered.

Findings that may be suggestive of unsatisfactory progress

Fetal condition

Fetal heart rate abnormalities (less than 100 beats/minute or more than 180 beats/minute heard before or after a contraction).

- change maternal position
- assess state of cervical dilatation
- continue to closely monitor fetal heart rate patterns
- check for positions or presentations in labour other than occiput anterior with a well-flexed vertex
- closely monitor progress of labour with use of partograph.

Maternal condition

- An increase in pulse rate. The woman may be dehydrated or in pain:
  - ☐ Ensure adequate hydration via oral or IV routes and provide adequate support/analgesia.
  - ☐ Check temperature for fever.
- Hypotension:
  - ☐ Change maternal position to lateral position.
  - ☐ If associated with haemorrhage: refer to management of obstetric haemorrhage (see **Module 5**).
- Acetone in urine (ketosis): the woman may be dehydrated: correct the hydration orally or IV.

Diagnosis of unsatisfactory progress of labour

Findings	Diagnosis
Cervix not dilated No palpable contractions/infrequent contractions	False labour
Cervix not dilated beyond 4 cm after 8 hours of regular contractions	Prolonged latent phase
Cervical dilatation to the right of the alert line on the partograph	Prolonged active phase
Secondary arrest of cervical dilatation and descent of presenting part in presence of good contractions; presenting part with large caput, third-degree moulding, cervix poorly applied to presenting part, oedematous cervix, ballooning of lower uterine segment, formation of retraction band, maternal and fetal distress	Obstructed labour with cephalopelvic disproportion
Less than three contractions in 10 minutes, each lasting 40 seconds or less	Inadequate uterine activity
Presentation other than cephalic with occiput anterior Cervix fully dilated and woman has urge to push but there is no descent after pushing	Malpresentation or malposition Prolonged expulsive phase Prolonged second stage if no delivery after 30 minutes pushing in a multiparous woman and after 60 minutes pushing in a primiparous woman

Management of unsatisfactory progress

False labour
- Examine for:
  - ☐ urinary tract infection
  - ☐ rupture of membranes.
- Treat accordingly.
- If none of these are present, discharge the woman.

Prolonged latent phase
- If a woman has been in the latent phase for more than 8 hours and there is little sign of progress, reassess the situation by assessing the cervix.
- Review the diagnosis of labour.
- If there has been a change in cervical effacement/dilatation, consider:
  - ☐ rupturing the membranes
  - ☐ inducing labour with oxytocin or prostaglandins.
- Reassess every 4 hours.

Prolonged active phase
- If there are no signs of cephalopelvic disproportion or obstruction:
  - ☐ rupture the membranes
  - ☐ assess uterine contractions.

- If uterine contractions are inadequate, consider augmentation.
- Encourage mobility.

Cephalopelvic disproportion

- If cephalopelvic disproportion is confirmed, deliver by caesarean section.
- If the fetus is dead, deliver by craniotomy if the operator is proficient.

Obstruction

- If the fetus is alive and the cervix fully dilated and head is at 0 station and is less than two-fifths palpable abdominally, deliver by vacuum extraction.
- If the fetus is alive but the cervix is not fully dilated, or if the fetal head is too high for vacuum extraction, deliver by caesarean section.
- If the fetus is dead, deliver by craniotomy.
- If the operator is not proficient in craniotomy, deliver by caesarean section.

Inadequate uterine activity

- If contractions are inefficient and cephalopelvic disproportion has been excluded:
  - ☐ rupture the membranes
  - ☐ augment labour with oxytocin.
- Reassess progress by vaginal examination 2 hours after a good contraction pattern is established.
- If no progress in 2 hours, deliver by caesarean section.

Prolonged expulsive phase

- If malpresentation and obvious obstruction have been excluded:
  - ☐ augment labour with oxytocin
  - ☐ change maternal position.

If there is no descent with augmentation:

- If the head is not more than two-fifths palpable above the symphysis pubis or the leading edge of the fetal head is at 0 station, deliver by vacuum extraction.
- If the head is more than two-fifths above the symphysis pubis or the leading bony edge of the fetal head is above −2 station, deliver by caesarean section.

Caesarean section

Doctors, midwives and theatre staff work together in a team to carry out this procedure.

[!] **Review indications. Ensure that vaginal delivery is not possible.**

Preparation: midwife

1. Tell the woman (and her support person) what is going to be done, listen to her, respond attentively to her questions and concerns and obtain informed consent.

2.   Examine the woman, assess her condition and examine the medical record for information and completeness.

3.   Check the fetal heart.

4.   Obtain blood for haemoglobin and blood type and crossmatch 2 units of blood.

5.   Set up an IV line and infuse 500 cc of IV fluids (normal saline or Ringer lactate).

6.   Give premedication including:
   ○   atropine 0.6 mg IM (or IV if in theatre)
   ○   magnesium trisilicate 300 mg.

7.   Help the woman to put on a gown and cap.

Preparation: scrub nurse

1.   Prepare the necessary equipment.

2.   Put on theatre clothes, protective footwear, cap, facemask, protective eyeglasses and a plastic apron.

3.   Perform a surgical hand scrub for 3–5 minutes and dry each hand on a separate sterile towel.

4.   Put on a sterile gown and put sterile surgical gloves on both hands.

5.   Ensure that the instruments and supplies are available and arrange them on a sterile tray or in a high-level disinfected container.

6.   Conduct an instrument and swab count and ask an assistant to note on board.

Preparation: doctor

1.   Examine the woman, assess her condition and examine the medical record for information and completeness.

2.   Check the fetal heart.

3.   Tell the woman (and her support person) what is going to be done, listen to her, respond attentively to her questions and concerns. Obtain informed consent if not already done so.

4.   Evaluate anaesthetic options:
   ○   general anaesthesia
   ○   local anaesthesia
   ○   spinal anaesthesia.

Pre-procedure tasks

1.   Put on theatre clothes, protective footwear, cap, facemask, protective eyeglasses and a plastic apron.

2.   Perform a surgical hand scrub for 3–5 minutes and dry each hand on a separate sterile towel.

3.   Put on a sterile gown and put high-level disinfected or sterile surgical gloves on both hands (double glove).

4.   Ensure that an assistant is scrubbed and dressed and that there is a midwife to receive the baby.

Preparing the woman

1.   Tilt operating table to the left or place a pillow under the woman's right lower back.

2.   Ensure that the woman has been anaesthetised and that the anaesthetic has taken full effect.

3.   Catheterise the woman.

4.   Apply antiseptic solution to the incision site and surrounding area three times. Allow to dry.

5.   Drape the abdomen, leaving the surgical area exposed and then drape the woman.

Procedure

1.   Ask the instrument nurse to stand with the instrument tray on the side opposite to you toward the foot of the woman.

2.   If you are right-handed, stand on the right side of the woman and ask the assistant to stand on the left side of the woman. If you are left-handed, it is easier to deliver the baby if you stand on the left side of the woman and the assistant on the right side.

3.   Make a midline vertical incision below the umbilicus to the pubic hair (or Pfannenstiel's incision – two fingers above the symphysis pubis), through the skin and to the level of the fascia.

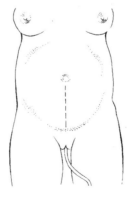

4.   Clamp any significant bleeding points with artery forceps and tie off the vessels with plain 0 catgut or polyglycolic (Vicryl® 2-0) or cauterise the tissue.

5.   Make a 2–3 cm vertical incision in the fascia (or transverse incision if using Pfannenstiel's incision).

6. Hold the fascia edge with forceps and lengthen the incision up and down (or left and right for Pfannenstiel) using scissors.

7. Use fingers or scissors to separate the rectus muscle.

8. Use fingers (or lift with forceps and open with scissors after checking no abdominal content in fold) to make an opening in the peritoneum near the umbilicus. Use scissors to lengthen the incision up and down in order to see the entire uterus.

9. Place a bladder retractor over the pubic bone.

10. Use forceps to pick up the loose peritoneum covering the anterior surface of the lower uterine segment and incise with scissors.

11. Extend the incision by placing the scissors between the uterus and the loose serosa and cutting about 3 cm on each side in a transverse fashion. Open this incision wider using fingers and move the bladder downwards carefully using fingers or a swab.

12. Replace the bladder retractor over the pubic bone to retract the bladder downward. Determine if a high vertical incision in the uterus is indicated rather than a lower uterine incision:
    ○ an inaccessible lower segment due to dense adhesions from previous section
    ○ transverse lie (with baby's back down) for which a lower uterine segment incision cannot be safely performed
    ○ large fibroids over the lower segment
    ○ carcinoma of the cervix
    ○ prematurity where the lower segment is not yet big enough.

13. Use a scalpel to make a 3-cm transverse incision in the lower segment of the uterus. It should be about 1 cm below the level where the vesico-uterine serosa was incised to bring the bladder down.

14. Widen the incision by placing a finger at each edge and gently pulling upward and laterally at the same time.

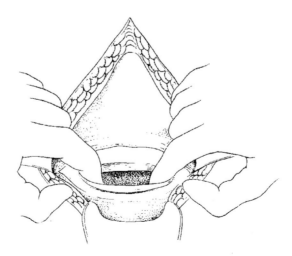

15. If it is necessary to extend the incision, do so using scissors instead of fingers to avoid extension into the uterine vessels. Make a crescent-shaped incision.

16. If the membranes are intact, rupture them. Ask the assistant to suction the liquid.

Delivering the newborn

1. Place one hand inside the uterine cavity between the uterus and the fetal head.

2. With your fingers, grasp and flex the head.

3. Gently lift the fetal head through the incision, taking care not to extend the incision down toward the cervix.

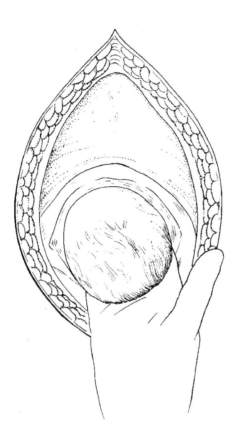

4. With the other hand, gently press on the abdomen over the top of the uterus to help deliver the head (and/or ask the assistant to give fundal pressure).

5. If the fetal head is deep in the pelvis or vagina, ask an assistant (not the scrubbed nurse) to put on sterile gloves to push the head up through the vagina from below. Then lift and deliver the head.

6. Ask the anaesthetist-nurse or assistant to check the blood pressure and give ergometrine 0.2 mg IV/IM if the blood pressure is less than 160/110. If blood pressure is 160/110 or higher, give oxytocin 20 units in 1 litre IV at 60 drops/minute for 2 hours.

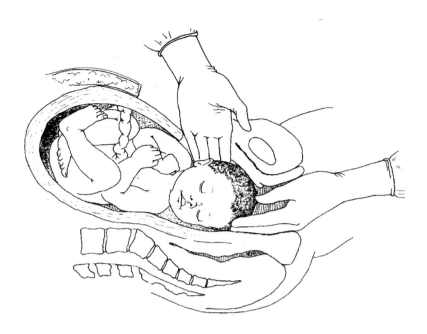

7.   Deliver the shoulders and body.

8.   Clamp the cord at two points and cut it.

9.   Hand the newborn to midwife or assistant.

10. Ask an assistant to give a single dose of prophylactic antibiotics, for example:
     ○ ampicillin 2 g IV

     OR

     ○ cefazolin 1 g IV

     OR

     ○ metronidazole 1 g IV.

11. Deliver the placenta by cord traction or manually.

12. Quickly inspect the placenta for completeness and abnormalities. Dilate cervix from above if necessary.

13. Swab out the uterus with a sterile swab to ensure no remnants of membranes and/or placental tissue.

Closing the uterine incision and abdomen

1.   Grasp the edges and corners of the uterine incision with Green Armytage clamps or ring forceps. Make sure that the clamp on the lower edge of the incision is separate from the bladder. Make sure that you have clearly identified the corners of the uterine incision.

2.   Identify again the corners and suture and tie them separately using 0 chromic catgut or polyglycolic so they are secure. Place a clamp on the end of the suture for easy reference.

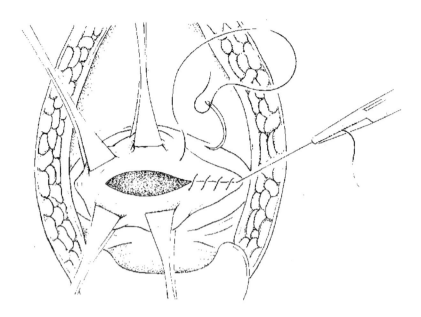

3. Repair the rest of the uterine incision, starting at the corner furthest away from you using a continuous locking stitch of 0 chromic catgut or polyglycolic suture. Take care not to touch the needle with fingers and use toothed forceps.

4. Secure haemostasis with a second layer of continuous suture taking care to invert any endometrium. Ensure haemostasis is complete. If there is any further bleeding from the incision site, close with figure-of-eight sutures.

5. Ensure the uterus is well contracted. If uterus not well contracted ask for a continuous infusion of 40 units oxytocin in 1 litre of saline or Ringer lactate to be given over the next 4–6 hours.

6. Ask the assistant to conduct an instrument and swab count and report back.

7. Before closing the abdomen, check for injury to the bladder. If the bladder has been injured, there will be fresh blood in the urine. Identify the extent of the injury and repair it.

8. Identify the end of the fascia at the upper and lower ends of the incision using Kocher's forceps. Place a clamp midway on either side of the incision. Close the fascia using a continuous 0 chromic catgut or polyglycolic suture ensuring there is no gap at either end.

9. If there are signs of infection, pack the subcutaneous tissue with gauze and place loose 0 catgut (or polyglycolic) sutures. Close the skin with a delayed closure after the infection has cleared.

10. If there are no signs of infection:
    ○ use a toothed dissecting forceps and a round needle threaded with plain catgut in a needle holder to place interrupted sutures to bring the fat layer together, if necessary.

○ use a toothed dissecting forceps and a cutting needle in a needle holder with 3-0 nylon (or silk) to place interrupted mattress sutures about 2 cm apart to bring the skin layer together.

11. Ensure there is no bleeding, clean the wound with gauze moistened in antiseptic solution and apply a sterile dressing.

12. Evacuate clots from vagina using forceps and swab and put on sterile pad.

13. Assist in getting woman off operating table.

Midwife's role in receiving the baby

1. Check resuscitation equipment is in working order and ensure radiant warmer is switched on and a good light is available.

2. Scrub up once the knife is to the skin.

3. Hold sterile cloth to receive the baby.

4. Carry the baby to the resuscitation area and rapidly dry him or her.

5. Wrap the baby in a clean dry cloth; simultaneously assess the Apgar score at 1 minute.

6. Respond to the need for resuscitation, as assessed.

7. Apply cord clamp and shorten cord stump using sterile equipment.

8. Label the baby. Record time of birth.

9. Keep the baby warm and in a safe environment.

10. Inform parents of baby's condition: keep mother and baby together.

Post-procedure tasks: doctor

1. Write notes of the operation, postoperative observations and management instructions.

2. Assess the woman before she is transferred out of the recovery area.

3. Check the woman on the ward daily or as frequently as necessary.

4. Discuss the reasons for the caesarean section, family planning and future pregnancies before discharge.

Post-procedure tasks: scrub-nurse

1. Dispose of needles and syringes: flush needle and syringe with 0.5% chlorine solution three times, then place in a puncture-proof container.

2. Remove gown and then immerse both gloved hands in 0.5% chlorine solution.

3. Remove gloves by turning them inside out. Dispose of gloves by placing them in a leakproof container or plastic bag.

4. Use antiseptic hand rub or wash hands thoroughly with soap and water and dry with a clean, dry cloth or air dry.

Postoperative care: midwife

1. **Immediate postoperative care: position** in left lateral 'recovery position'; maintain clear airway.

2. **Observations:**
   ○ pulse: every 15 minutes initially
   ○ blood pressure: every 15 minutes initially
   ○ respiration rate: every 15 minutes initially
   ○ check bleeding:
     – from the wound every 30 minutes
     – vaginally every 30 minutes
   ○ check uterus is contracted: every 30 minutes.

3. Maintain prescribed **IV infusion.**

4. **Assess level of pain** and provide adequate pain relief.

5. **Assist mother to place baby at breast** if mother is breastfeeding.

Care in the postnatal ward

■ Observations: continue 4-hourly temperature, pulse and respiration rate and BP for first 48 hours.

■ Ensure adequate pain relief.

■ Monitor urinary output.

■ Ensure good hydration:
  □ ensure adequate IV infusion in first 24 hours
  □ start taking sips of water within 24 hours
  □ gradually increase to food, if no nausea, after 24 hours.

■ Encourage the mother to take deep breaths and move her legs while in bed.

■ Help the mother to get out of bed as soon as possible to aid circulation.

■ Manage wound care as local protocol.

■ Assist with maintaining good hygiene practices and regular changing of sanitary pads.

■ Keep mother and baby together.

■ Support breastfeeding practices.

Prior to going home

■ Discuss reasons for caesarean section, family planning and future pregnancies and delivery before discharge.

■ Discuss need for rest, nutrition and hygiene for mother.

■ Discuss newborn care and good feeding practices.

■ Schedule appointment for postpartum care.

Guide for laparotomy for ruptured uterus

Preparation and pre-procedure tasks: as for **caesarean section**.

Ensure that a **laparotomy tray** is used.

Delivery procedure

1. Open the abdomen as for caesarean section but use a midline abdominal incision.

2. Deliver the newborn and placenta.

3. Ask the anaesthetist to infuse oxytocin 40 units in 1 litre normal saline or Ringer lactate at 60 drops/minute.

4. Check for uterine contractions. After the uterus contracts, ask the anaesthetist to reduce the oxytocin infusion rate to 20 drops/minute.

5. Lift the uterus out of the pelvis and examine the front, back and sides of the uterus.

6. Consider repair of the uterus if:
   ○ there is a wish for future pregnancy
   ○ the woman will have access to emergency obstetric care for her next pregnancy
   ○ it is surgically feasible to conduct repair without damage to the bladder or ureter
   ○ the edges of the tear are clearly identified and not necrotic.

Repair of uterus

1. Hold the bleeding edges of the uterus with Green Armytage clamps (or ring forceps).

2. Separate the urinary bladder from the lower uterine segment by sharp and blunt dissection.

3. Determine if the tear is through the cervix and vagina or laterally through the uterine artery or if there is a broad ligament haematoma and repair as necessary.

4. Repair the uterine tear using continuous locking sutures with 0 chromic catgut (or polyglycolic) suture, ensuring the ureter is not included in a stitch.

5. Place a second layer of sutures if the bleeding is not controlled or if the upper segment of the uterus is involved in the rupture.

6. Check the fallopian tubes and ovaries. If tubal ligation was requested, perform the procedure.

7. If there is bleeding, control by clamping with long artery forceps and ligating. If the bleeding points are deep, use figure-of-eight sutures.

8. Place an abdominal drain:
   ○ make a stab incision in the lower abdomen about 3–4 cm away from the edge of the midline incision, just below the level of the anterior superior iliac spine
   ○ insert a long clamp through the incision

○ grasp the end of the abdominal drain and bring this end out through the incision

○ ensure that the peritoneal end of the drain is in place and anchor the drain to the skin with nylon or silk suture.

9.   Ensure that there is no bleeding and remove any blood clots. If there is a haematoma, drain it.

10.   Before closing the abdomen, check for injury to the bladder. If the bladder has been injured, identify the extent of the injury and repair it.

11.   Close the abdomen as for caesarean section.

Post-procedure care

1.   Transfer the woman to the recovery area. Do not leave the woman unattended until the effects of the anaesthesia have worn off.

2.   Write notes of the operation, postoperative observations and management instructions.

3.   Assess the woman before she is transferred out of the recovery area.

4.   Once the woman has woken fully from the anaesthesia, explain what was found at surgery and what procedures have been done.

5.   Ensure that the woman has written postoperative instructions (such as awareness of complications and warning signs, when to return to work) and necessary medications before discharge.

6.   Tell her when to return if follow up is needed and that she can return anytime she has concerns.

7.   If tubal ligation was not performed, discuss reproductive goals, provide counselling on prognosis for fertility and, if appropriate, provide family planning. If the woman wishes to have more children, advise her to have an elective caesarean section for future pregnancies.

Subtotal (supracervical) hysterectomy

1.   Lift the uterus out of the abdomen and gently pull to maintain traction.

2.   Doubly clamp and cut the round ligaments with scissors. Clamp and cut the pedicles, but ligate after the uterine arteries are secured to save time.

3.   From the edge of the cut round ligament, open the anterior leaf of the broad ligament.

4.   Incise to:
   ○ the point where the bladder peritoneum is reflected onto the lower uterine surface in the midline

   OR

   ○ the incised peritoneum at a caesarean section.

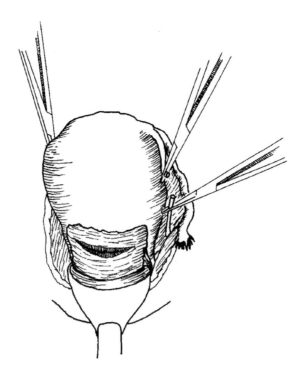

5. Use two fingers to push the posterior leaf of the broad ligament forward, just under the tube and ovary, near the uterine edge. Make a hole the size of a finger in the broad ligament, using scissors. Doubly clamp and cut the tube, the ovarian ligament and the broad ligament through the hole in the broad ligament.

[!] The ureters are close to the uterine vessels. The ureter must be identified and exposed to avoid injuring it during surgery or including it in a stitch.

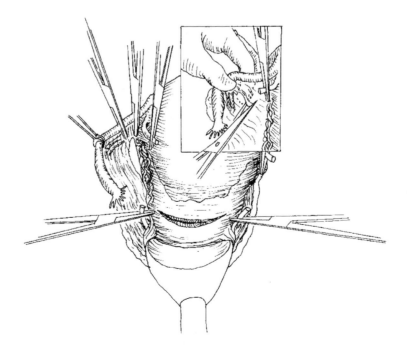

6. Divide the posterior leaf of the broad ligament downwards towards the uterosacral ligaments, using scissors.

7. Grasp the edge of the bladder flap with forceps or a small clamp. Using fingers or scissors, dissect the bladder downwards off of the lower uterine segment. Direct the pressure downwards but inwards toward the cervix and the lower uterine segment.

8. Locate the uterine artery and vein on each side of the uterus. Feel for the junction of the uterus and cervix.

9. Doubly clamp across the uterine vessels at a 90-degree angle on each side of the cervix. Cut and doubly ligate with 0 chromic catgut (or polyglycolic) suture.

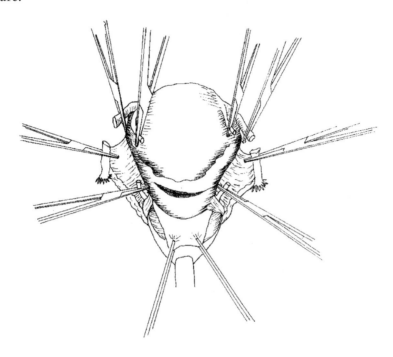

10. Observe carefully for any further bleeding. **If the uterine arteries are ligated correctly,** bleeding should stop and the uterus should look pale.

11. Return to the clamped pedicles of the round ligaments and tubo-ovarian ligaments and ligate them with 0 chromic catgut (or polyglycolic) suture.

12. Amputate the uterus above the level where the uterine arteries are ligated, using scissors.

13. Close the cervical stump with interrupted 2-0 or 3-0 chromic catgut (or polyglycolic) sutures.

14. Carefully inspect the cervical stump, leaves of the broad ligament and other pelvic floor structures for any bleeding.

15. **If slight bleeding persists or a clotting disorder is suspected,** place a drain through the abdominal wall. Do not place a drain through the cervical stump as this can cause postoperative infection.

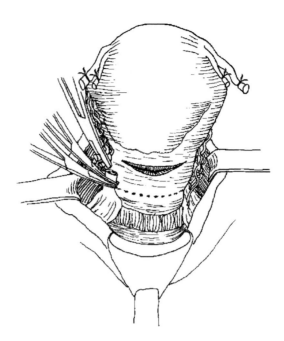

16. Ensure that there is no bleeding. Remove clots using a sponge.

17. In all cases, check for injury to the bladder. **If a bladder injury is identified,** repair the injury.

18. Close the fascia with continuous 0 chromic catgut (or polyglycolic) suture.

[!] There is no need to close the bladder peritoneum or the abdominal peritoneum.

19. If there are **signs of infection,** pack the subcutaneous tissue with gauze and place loose 0 catgut (or polyglycolic) sutures. Close the skin with a delayed closure after the infection has cleared.

20. If there are **no signs of infection,** close the skin with vertical mattress sutures of 3-0 nylon (or silk) and apply a sterile dressing.

Total hysterectomy

The following additional steps are required for total hysterectomy:

1. Push the bladder down to free the top 2 cm of the vagina.

2. Open the posterior leaf of the broad ligament.

3. Clamp, cut and ligate the uterosacral ligaments.

4. Clamp, cut and ligate the cardinal ligaments, which contain the descending branches of the uterine vessels. This is the critical step in the operation:
    ○ grasp the ligament vertically with a large-toothed clamp (such as Kocher)
    ○ place the clamp 5 mm lateral to the cervix and cut the ligament close to the cervix, leaving a stump medial to the clamp for safety
    ○ if the cervix is long, repeat the step two or three times as needed.

5. The upper 2 cm of the vagina should now be free of attachments.

6. Circumcise the vagina as near to the cervix as possible, clamping bleeding points as they appear.

7. Place haemostatic angle sutures, which include round, cardinal and uterosacral ligaments.

8. Place continuous sutures on the vaginal cuff to stop haemorrhage.

9. Close the abdomen (as above) after placing a drain in the extraperitoneal space near the stump of the cervix.

Postoperative care
- Review postoperative care principles.
- If there are **signs of infection** or the woman **currently has fever**, give a combination of antibiotics until she is fever-free for 48 hours:
  - ☐ ampicillin 2 g IV every 6 hours

    PLUS

  - ☐ gentamicin 5 mg/kg body weight IV every 24 hours

    PLUS

  - ☐ metronidazole 500 mg IV every 8 hours.
- Give appropriate analgesic drugs.
- If there are **no signs of infection**, remove the abdominal drain after 48 hours.
- Note that, especially with late presentation or diagnosis of ruptured uterus, abdominal distension can occur postoperatively with ileus, which may require nasogastric tube.

Symphysiotomy

Symphysiotomy results in temporary increase in pelvic diameter (up to 2 cm) by surgically dividing the ligaments of the symphysis under local anaesthesia.

This procedure should only be carried out in combination with vacuum extraction.

Risks
- Urethral and bladder injury.
- Infection.
- Pain.
- Long-term walking difficulty.

Indications
- Contracted pelvis/cephalopelvic disproportion.
- Vertex presentation.
- Prolonged second stage.
- Failure to descend after proper augmentation.

- Failure or anticipated failure or vacuum extraction alone.
- Breech presentation with entrapped head.

Conditions necessary for symphysiotomy

- Fetus is alive.
- Cervix is fully dilated.
- Fetal head is at –2 station or no more than three-fifths above the symphysis pubis.
- No over-riding of the head above the symphysis.
- Caesarean section is not feasible or immediately available.
- The provider is experienced and proficient in symphysiotomy.

Procedure

1. Provide emotional support and encouragement.

2. Use local infiltration with lignocaine.

3. Ask two assistants to support the woman's legs with her thighs and knees flexed. The thighs should be abducted no more than 45 degrees from the midline.

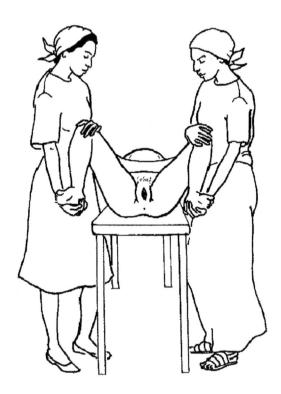

4. Perform a mediolateral episiotomy. If an episiotomy is already present, enlarge it to minimise stretching of the vaginal wall and urethra.

5. Infiltrate the anterior, superior and inferior aspects of the symphysis with lignocaine 0.5% solution.

[!] Aspirate (pull back on the plunger) to be sure that no vessel has been penetrated. If blood is returned in the syringe with aspiration, remove the needle. Recheck the position carefully and try again. Never inject if blood is aspirated: the woman can suffer convulsions and death if IV injection occurs.

6. At the conclusion of the set of injections, wait 2 minutes and then pinch the incision site with forceps. If the woman feels the pinch, wait 2 more minutes and then retest.

7. Insert a firm catheter to identify the urethra.

8. Apply antiseptic solution to the suprapubic skin.

9. Wearing sterile gloves, place an index finger into the vagina and push the catheter, with it the urethra, away from the midline.

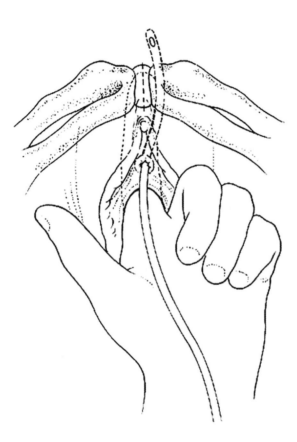

10. With the other hand, use a thick, firm-bladed scalpel to make a vertical stab incision over the symphysis.

11. Keeping to the midline, cut down through the cartilage joining the two pubic bones until the pressure of the scalpel blade is felt on the finger in the vagina.

12. Cut the cartilage downwards to the bottom of the symphysis, then rotate the blade and cut upwards to the top of the symphysis.

13. Once the symphysis has been divided though its whole length, the pubic bone will separate.

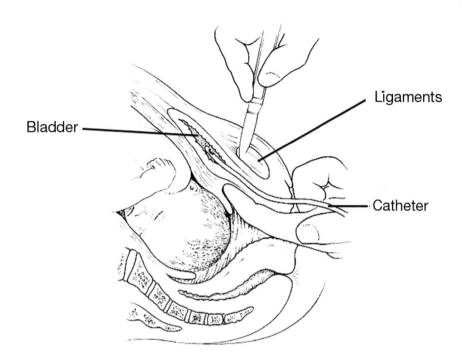

14. After separating the cartilage, remove the catheter to decrease urethral trauma.

15. Deliver the baby by vacuum extraction. Descent of the head causes the symphysis to separate 1–2 cm.

16. After delivery, catheterise the bladder with a self-retaining bladder catheter.

17. There is no need to close the stab incision, unless there is bleeding.

Post-procedure care

1. If there are signs of infection or the woman currently has fever, give a combination of antibiotics until she is fever-free for 48 hours:
   ○ ampicillin 2 g IV every 6 hours

      PLUS

   ○ gentamicin 5 mg/kg body weight IV every 24 hours

      PLUS
   ○ metronidazole 500 mg IV every 8 hours.

2. Give appropriate analgesic drugs.

3. Apply elastic strapping across the front of the pelvis from one iliac crest to the other, to stabilise the symphysis and to reduce pain.

4. Leave the catheter in the bladder for a minimum of 5 days.

5. Encourage the woman to drink plenty of fluids to ensure a good urinary output.

6. Encourage bed rest for 7 days after discharge from hospital.

7. Encourage the woman to begin to walk with assistance when she is ready to do so.

8. If long-term walking difficulties and pain are reported (these occur with 2% of cases), treat with physiotherapy.

Craniotomy

In certain cases of obstructed labour with fetal death, reduction in the size of the fetal head by craniotomy makes a vaginal delivery possible and avoids the risks associated with caesarean delivery.

Preparation
■ Provide emotional support and encouragement.
■ If necessary, give diazepam IV slowly or use a pudendal block.
■ Apply antiseptic solution to the vagina.
■ Perform an episiotomy, if required.

Procedure
Cephalic presentation
1. Make a cruciate (cross-shaped) incision on the scalp.

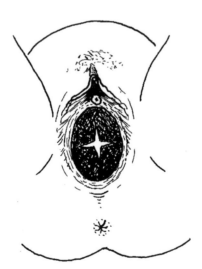

2. Open the cranial vault at the lowest and most central bony point with a craniotome (or large-pointed scissors or a heavy scalpel). In face presentation, perforate the orbits.

3. Insert the craniotome into the fetal cranium and fragment the intracranial contents.

4. Grasp the edges of the skull with several heavy-toothed forceps (such as Kocher) and apply traction in the axis of the birth canal.

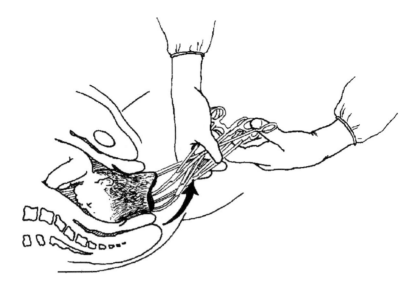

5. As the head descends, pressure from the bony pelvis will cause the skull to collapse, decreasing the cranial diameter.

6. After delivery, examine the woman carefully and repair any tears to the cervix and vagina and repair the episiotomy.

7. Leave a self-retaining catheter in place until it is confirmed that there is no bladder injury.

8. Ensure adequate fluid intake and urinary output.

Breech presentation with entrapped head

Note that symphysiotomy may also be considered.

1. Make an incision through the skin at the base of the neck.

2. Insert a craniotome (or large-pointed scissors or a heavy scalpel) through the incision and tunnel subcutaneously to reach the occiput.

3. Perforate the occiput and open the gap as widely as possible.

4. Apply traction on the trunk to collapse the skull as the head descends.

Module 7
Sepsis

Aim

- To learn to recognise sepsis.
- To practise an effective response to a woman with sepsis.

Recognition

- Fever: temperature 38°C or above.
- Warm extremities.
- Fast breathing.
- Increased heart rate: mother (and fetus).
- Low BP.
- Altered mental state: confused, restless.
- Septic shock.

[!] Someone in septic shock may not have a raised temperature (fever). There is a pounding pulse and warm extremities.

Management

- Start IV and if the woman is conscious, encourage increased fluid intake by mouth.
- Use a fan and/or tepid sponging to help decrease temperature.
- If shock is suspected, begin antibiotic (and antimalarial) treatment at once, intravenously.
- Treat the cause.

Sepsis during pregnancy and labour

Recognising sepsis

- A woman has a fever (temperature 38°C or more) during pregnancy or labour.
- If there are palpable contractions and bloodstained mucus discharge, suspect preterm labour as a complication of sepsis and begin treatment immediately.

Causes

Causes of fever during pregnancy and labour

Presenting symptoms and signs		Probable diagnosis
Usually present	**Sometimes present**	
Dysuria Increased frequency and urgency of urination	Retropubic/suprapubic pain Abdominal pain	Cystitis
Dysuria Spiking fever/chills Increased frequency and urgency of urination Abdominal pain	Retropubic/suprapubic pain Loin pain/tenderness Tenderness in rib cage Anorexia Nausea/vomiting	Acute pyelonephritis
Foul-smelling vaginal discharge in early pregnancy Fever Tender uterus	Lower abdominal pain Rebound tenderness Prolonged bleeding Purulent cervical discharge	Septic abortion
Fever/chills Foul-smelling watery discharge History of ruptured membranes Abdominal pain	History of rupture of membranes/loss of fluid Tender uterus Rapid/absent fetal heart rate Light vaginal bleeding	Amnionitis
Fever Difficulty in breathing Productive cough Chest pain	Consolidation Congested throat Rapid breathing Rhonchi/rales	Pneumonia
Fever Chills/rigors Headache Muscle/joint pain	Enlarged spleen	Malaria (uncomplicated)
Symptoms and signs of malaria Coma Anaemia	Convulsions Jaundice	Severe malaria (complicated)
Fever Headache Dry cough Malaise Anorexia Enlarged spleen	Confusion Stupor	Typhoid fever
Fever Malaise Anorexia Nausea Jaundice Enlarged liver	Muscle/joint pain Urticaria Enlarged spleen	Hepatitis

Cystitis and pyelonephritis

Tests:

- A dipstick leukocyte esterase test can be used to detect white blood cells and a nitrate reductase test can be used to detect nitrites.
- Microscopy of urine specimen may show white cells in clumps, bacteria and sometimes red cells.

Treatment for cystitis – infection of the bladder

Treat with antibiotics:

- amoxicillin 500 mg by mouth three times/day for 3 days.

    OR

- trimethoprim/sulfamethoxazole 1 tablet (160/800 mg) by mouth two times/day for 3 days.

If infection recurs two or more times:

- Check urine culture and sensitivity, if available, and treat with an antibiotic appropriate for the organism.
- For prophylaxis against further infections, give antibiotics by mouth once daily for the remainder of pregnancy and 2 weeks postpartum.

Give:

- trimethoprim/sulfamethoxazole 1 tablet (160/800 mg)

    OR

- amoxicillin 250 mg.

Treatment for acute pyelonephritis

Acute pyelonephritis is an acute infection of the upper urinary tract, mainly of the renal pelvis, which may also involve renal parenchyma.

If shock is present or suspected, initiate immediate treatment.

Treat with IV antibiotics until the woman is fever-free for 48 hours:

- ampicillin 2 g IV every 6 hours

    PLUS

- gentamicin 5 mg/kg body weight IV every 24 hours.

Once the woman is fever-free for 48 hours, give amoxicillin 1 g by mouth three times/day to complete 14 days of treatment.

[!] **Clinical response is expected within 48 hours. If there is no clinical response in 72 hours, think about other possible causes of the fever and whether the antibiotic coverage is sufficient.**

For prophylaxis against further infections, give antibiotics by mouth once daily at bedtime for the remainder of pregnancy and for 2 weeks postpartum.

Give:

■ trimethoprim/sulfamethoxazole 1 tablet (160/800 mg)

OR

■ amoxicillin 250 mg.

Ensure adequate hydration by mouth or IV.

Give paracetamol 500 mg by mouth as needed for pain and to lower temperature.

Malaria

Symptomatic falciparum malaria in pregnant women may cause severe disease and death if not recognised and treated early.

When malaria presents as an acute illness with fever, it cannot be reliably distinguished from other causes of fever on clinical grounds only.

Malaria should always be considered together with infection as the most likely causes in a pregnant woman with fever.

Tests:

■ If facilities for testing are not available, begin therapy with antimalarial drugs based on clinical suspicion (such as headache, fever, joint pain).
■ Where available, perform microscopy of a thick and thin blood film:
   ☐ thick blood film is more sensitive at detecting parasites (absence of parasites does not rule out malaria)
   ☐ thin blood film helps to identify the parasite species.

Typhoid

Give ampicillin 1 g by mouth four times/day OR give amoxicillin 1 g by mouth three times/day for 14 days. Alternative therapy will depend on local sensitivity patterns.

Hepatitis

Provide supportive therapy and observe.

Sepsis after delivery

Recognition
A woman has a fever (temperature 38°C or more) occurring more than 24 hours after delivery.

Causes of fever after childbirth

Presenting symptom and other symptoms and signs		Probable diagnosis
Usually present	**Sometimes present**	
Fever/chills Lower abdominal pain Purulent, foul-smelling lochia Tender uterus	Vaginal bleeding Shock	Endometritis
Lower abdominal pain and distension Persistent spiking fever/chills Tender uterus Bowel symptoms, such as diarrhoea	Poor response to antibiotics Swelling in adnexa or pouch of Douglas Pus obtained upon culdocentesis	Pelvic abscess
Low-grade fever/chills Lower abdominal pain Absent bowel sounds	Rebound tenderness Abdominal distension Anorexia Nausea/vomiting Shock	Peritonitis
Breast pain and tenderness 3–5 days after delivery	Hard, enlarged breasts Both breasts affected	Breast engorgement
Breast pain and tenderness Discoloured, wedge-shaped area on breast 3–4 weeks after delivery	Inflammation preceded by engorgement Usually only one breast affected	Mastitis
Firm, very tender breast Overlying discoloration	Fluctuant swelling in breast Draining pus	Breast abscess
Unusually tender wound with bloody or serous discharge	Slight discoloration extending beyond edge of incision	Wound abscess, wound seroma or wound haematoma
Painful and tender wound Discoloration and oedema beyond edge of incision	Hardened wound Purulent discharge Reddened area around wound	Wound cellulitis
Spiking fever despite antibiotics	Calf muscle tenderness	Deep vein thrombosis
Fever Decreased breath sounds	Typically occurs postoperatively	Atelectasis

Endometritis
Endometritis is infection of the uterus after delivery and is a major cause of maternal death.

Delayed or inadequate treatment of endometritis may result in pelvic abscess, peritonitis, septic shock, deep vein thrombosis, pulmonary embolism, chronic pelvic infection with recurrent pelvic pain and dyspareunia, tubal blockage and infertility.

Check haemoglobin and give blood transfusion if necessary.

Give a combination of IV antibiotics until the woman is fever-free for 48 hours:

■ ampicillin 2 g IV every 6 hours

PLUS

■ gentamicin 5 mg/kg body weight IV every 24 hours

PLUS

■ metronidazole 500 mg IV every 8 hours.

If fever is still present 72 hours after initiating antibiotics:

■ re-evaluate and consider other causes of fever such as malaria
■ consider if antibiotic cover sufficient
■ consider HIV status.

If retained placental fragments are suspected, give anaesthesia and perform a digital exploration of the uterus to remove clots and large pieces. Use ovum forceps or a large curette if required.

If there is no improvement with conservative measures and there are signs of general peritonitis (fever, rebound tenderness, abdominal pain), perform a laparotomy to drain the pus. If the uterus is necrotic and septic, perform subtotal hysterectomy.

Pelvic abscess

Give a combination of antibiotics before draining the abscess and continue until the woman is fever-free for 48 hours:

■ ampicillin 2 g IV every 6 hours

PLUS

■ gentamicin 5 mg/kg body weight IV every 24 hours

PLUS

■ metronidazole 500 mg IV every 8 hours.

If the abscess is fluctuant in the cul-de-sac, drain the pus through the cul-de-sac. If the spiking fever continues, perform a laparotomy.

Peritonitis

Insert nasogastric tube. Start an IV infusion and infuse IV fluids.

Give a combination of antibiotics until the woman is fever-free for 48 hours:

■ ampicillin 2 g IV every 6 hours

PLUS

■ gentamicin 5 mg/kg body weight IV every 24 hours

PLUS

■ metronidazole 500 mg IV every 8 hours.

If necessary, perform laparotomy for peritoneal lavage (wash-out).

Breast engorgement

Breast engorgement is an exaggeration of the lymphatic and venous engorgement that occurs prior to lactation. It is not the result of over distension of the breast with milk.

Breastfeeding

If the woman is breastfeeding and the baby is not able to suckle, encourage the woman to express milk.

If the woman is breastfeeding and the baby is able to suckle:

■ encourage the woman to breastfeed more frequently, using both breasts at each feeding
■ show the woman how to hold the baby and help it attach.

Relief measures before feeding may include:

■ Apply warm compresses to the breasts just before breastfeeding
■ Encourage the woman to take a warm shower
■ Massage the woman's neck and back
■ Have the woman express some milk manually prior to breastfeeding to soften the nipple area to help the baby latch on properly and easily.

Relief measures after feeding may include:

■ Support breasts with a binder or brassiere.
■ Apply cold compress to the breasts between feedings to reduce swelling and pain.
■ Give paracetamol 500 mg by mouth as needed.
■ Follow up 3 days after initiating management to ensure response.

If the woman is not breastfeeding:

■ Support breasts with a binder or brassiere.
■ Apply cold compresses to the breasts to reduce swelling and pain.
■ Avoid massaging or applying heat to the breasts.
■ Avoid stimulating the nipples.
■ Give paracetamol 500 mg by mouth as needed.

Breast infection
Mastitis
Treat with antibiotics:

■ cloxacillin 500 mg by mouth four times/day for 10 days

OR

■ erythromycin 250 mg by mouth three times/day for 10 days.

Encourage the woman to:

■ continue breastfeeding
■ support breasts with a binder or brassiere
■ apply cold compresses to the breasts between feedings to reduce swelling and pain

Give paracetamol 500 mg by mouth as needed.

Follow up in 3 days to ensure response.

Breast abscess
Treat with antibiotics:

■ cloxacillin 500 mg by mouth four times/day for 10 days

   OR

■ erythromycin 250 mg by mouth three times/day for 10 days.
■ Drain the abscess.
■ General anaesthesia (e.g. ketamine) is usually required.
■ Make the incision radially, extending from near the alveolar margin towards the periphery of the breast to avoid injury to the milk ducts.
■ Wearing sterile gloves, use a finger or tissue forceps to break up the pockets of pus.
■ Loosely pack the cavity with gauze.
■ Remove the gauze pack after 24 hours and replace with a smaller gauze pack.
■ If there is still pus in the cavity, place a small gauze pack in the cavity and bring the edge out through the wound as a wick to facilitate drainage of any remaining pus.
■ Encourage the woman to:
   □ continue breastfeeding even when there is collection of pus
   □ support breasts with a binder or brassiere
   □ apply cold compresses to the breasts between feedings to reduce swelling and pain.
■ Give paracetamol 500 mg by mouth as needed
■ Follow up in 3 days to ensure response.

Infection of perineal and abdominal wounds
If there is pus or fluid, open and drain the wound, remove infected skin or subcutaneous sutures and debride the wound. Do not remove fascial sutures.

If there is an abscess without cellulitis, antibiotics are not required.

Place a damp dressing in the wound and have the woman return to change the dressing every 24 hours.

Advise the woman on the need for good hygiene and to wear clean pads or cloths that she changes often.

If infection is superficial and does not involve deep tissues, monitor for development of an abscess and give a combination of antibiotics:

- ampicillin 500 mg by mouth four times/day for 5 days

  PLUS

- metronidazole 400 mg by mouth three times/day for 5 days.

If the infection is deep, involves muscles and is causing necrosis (necrotising fasciitis), give a combination of antibiotics until necrotic tissue has been removed and the woman is fever-free for 48 hours:

- penicillin G 2 million units IV every 6 hours

  PLUS

- gentamicin 5 mg/kg body weight IV every 24 hours

  PLUS

- metronidazole 500 mg IV every 8 hours.

Once the woman is fever-free for 48 hours, give:

- ampicillin 500 mg by mouth four times/day for 5 days

  PLUS

- metronidazole 400 mg by mouth three times/day for 5 days.

[!] Necrotising fasciitis requires wide surgical debridement. Perform secondary closure 2–4 weeks later, depending on resolution of infection.

Deep vein thrombosis
Commence heparin infusion.

Atelectasis
Encourage ambulation and deep breathing.

Give appropriate IV/IM antibiotics.

Give the first dose of antibiotic(s) before referral. If referral is delayed or not possible, continue antibiotics IM/IV for 48 hours after woman is fever-free.

Then give amoxicillin orally 500 mg 3 times daily until 7 days of treatment completed.

If signs persist or mother becomes weak or has abdominal pain postpartum, **refer urgently to hospital.**

Antibiotic treatment

Condition Antibiotics

Severe abdominal pain
Dangerous fever/very severe febrile disease
Complicated abortion
Uterine and fetal infection
	Three antibiotics:
	    ampicillin
	    gentamicin
	    metronidazole

Postpartum bleeding
        lasting > 24 hours
        occurring > 24 hours after delivery
Upper urinary tract infection
	Two antibiotics:
	    ampicillin
	    gentamicin

Pneumonia Manual removal of placenta/fragments Risk of uterine and fetal infection In labour > 24 hours	One antibiotic: ampicillin

Antibiotic	Preparation	Dosage/route	Frequency
Ampicillin	Vial containing 500 mg as powder: to be mixed with 2.5 ml sterile water	First 2 g IV/IM then 1 g	Every 6 hours
Gentamicin	Vial containing 40 mg/ml in 2 ml	80 mg IM	Every 8 hours
Metronidazole DO NOT GIVE IM	Vial containing 500 mg in 100 ml	500 mg or 100 ml IV infusion	Every 8 hours
Erythromycin (if allergic to ampicillin)	Vial containing 500 mg as powder	500 mg IV/IM	Every 6 hours

Module 8
Assisted delivery

Aim

- To recognise when it is necessary to assist delivery using vacuum extraction.
- To understand the principles of the use of vacuum extraction.
- To understand the basic principles of simple forceps delivery.
- To understand the principles underlying the repair of vaginal and perineal tears.

Vacuum extraction

Indications for vacuum extraction include:

- Prolonged second stage.
- Fetal distress in second stage.
- To expedite delivery (for example maternal exhaustion, placental abruption, cord prolapse at full dilatation).

Conditions necessary for vacuum extraction
- Cephalic (vertex) presentation.
- Cervix fully dilated.
- Fetal head at least at 0 station (at spines) or lower.
- Fetal head not more than two-fifths palpable above the symphysis pubis.
- Ruptured membranes.
- Adequate analgesia: pudendal block if possible and perineal infiltration.

Preparation
1. Prepare the necessary equipment.

2. Tell the woman (and her support person) what is going to be done, listen to her and respond attentively to her questions and concerns.

3. Provide continual emotional support

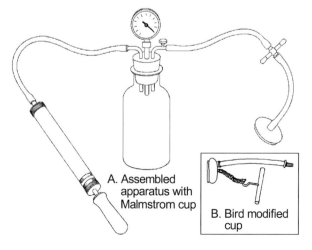

A. Assembled apparatus with Malmstrom cup

B. Bird modified cup

and reassurance, as feasible.

Pre-procedure tasks

1. Use antiseptic hand rub or wash hands thoroughly with soap and water and dry with a sterile cloth or air dry and put on gloves.

2. Drape the mother.

3. Clean the vulva with antiseptic solution.

4. Catheterise the bladder.

5. Check all connections on the vacuum extractor and test the vacuum on a gloved hand.

6. If possible, use a pudendal block.

Procedure

1. Assess the position of the fetal head by feeling the sagittal suture line and the

Landmarks of the fetal skull

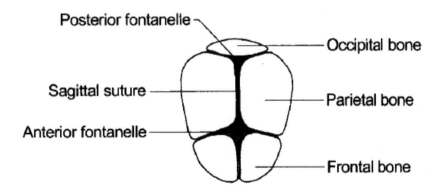

fontanelles.

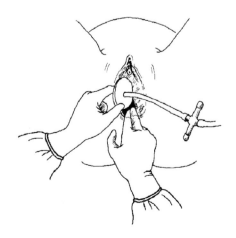

2. Identify the posterior fontanelle.

3. Between contractions, apply the largest cup that will fit, with the centre of the cup over the posterior fontanelle.

4. Perform an episiotomy, if necessary, for proper placement of the cup. If episiotomy is not necessary for placement of the cup, delay cutting the episiotomy until the head stretches the perineum or the perineum interferes with the axis of traction.

5. Check the application and ensure that there is no maternal soft tissue (cervix or vagina) within the rim of the cup.

6. Have the assistant create a vacuum of 0.2 kg/cm² (usually yellow colour) negative pressure with the pump and check the application of the cup. If necessary, release pressure and reapply cup.

7. Increase the vacuum to 0.8 kg/cm² (usually green colour) negative pressure and check the application of the cup.

8. After maximum negative pressure has been applied, start traction in the line of the pelvic axis and perpendicular to the cup.
   ○ If the fetal head is tilted to one side or not flexed well, traction should be directed in a line that will try to correct the tilt or deflexion of the head (that is, to one side or the other, not necessarily in the midline).

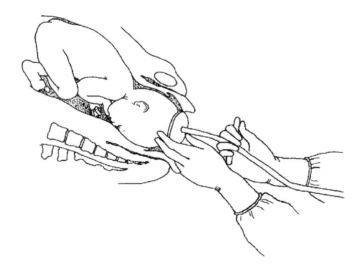

9. With each contraction, ask the mother to push and apply traction in a line perpendicular to the plane of the cup rim.
   ○ Place a gloved finger on the scalp next to the cup during traction to assess potential slippage and descent of the vertex.

[!] **Between each contraction check:**
   ○ **fetal heart rate**
   ○ **application of the cup**

Do not continue to pull if there is no contraction.

10. With progress, and in the absence of fetal distress, continue the 'guiding' pulls for a maximum of 30 minutes.

11. When the head has been delivered, release the vacuum, remove the cup and complete the birth of the newborn.

12. Perform active management of the third stage of labour to deliver the placenta:
    ○ 10 units oxytocin IM
    ○ controlled cord traction.

13. Check the birth canal for tears following childbirth and repair episiotomy.

Post-procedure tasks

1. Before removing gloves, dispose of waste materials in a leakproof container or plastic bag.

2. Use antiseptic hand rub or wash hands thoroughly with soap and water and dry with a clean, dry cloth or air dry.

3. Record the procedure and findings on woman's record.

Failed vacuum extraction

■ Classify a failed vacuum extraction if:
   □ fetal head does not advance with each pull
   □ fetus is undelivered after three pulls or after 30 minutes
   □ cup slips off the head twice at the proper direction of pull with a maximum negative pressure.
■ Every application should be considered a trial of vacuum extraction. Do not persist if there is no descent with every pull.
■ If vacuum extraction fails, perform a caesarean section.
■ Use vacuum extraction in combination with symphysiotomy only if this is accepted practice and the provider is competent in this procedure.

Forceps delivery

Indications for forceps delivery:

■ Aftercoming head of a breech.
■ Preference over vacuum extraction by attending doctor.

Preparation

1. Prepare the necessary equipment.

2. Tell the woman (and her support person) what is going to be done, listen to her and respond attentively to her questions and concerns.

3. Provide continual emotional support and reassurance, as feasible.

Conditions necessary for forceps delivery

- Vertex presentation or face presentation with chin-anterior or entrapped after-coming head in breech delivery.
- Cervix fully dilated.
- Fetal head at +2 or +3 station palpable or 0/5 (that is, not palpable) above the symphysis pubis.
- Ruptured membranes.
- Adequate analgesia: pudendal block if possible and perineal infiltration.

Pre-procedure tasks

1. Use antiseptic hand rub or wash hands thoroughly with soap and water and dry with a sterile cloth or air dry.

2. Put on sterile surgical gloves and drape the woman.

3. Clean the vulva with antiseptic solution.

4. Catheterise the bladder.

5. Assemble the forceps before application. Ensure that the parts fit together and lock well.

6. Lubricate the blades of the forceps with antiseptic gel.

7. If possible and time permits (fetal condition) use a pudendal block.

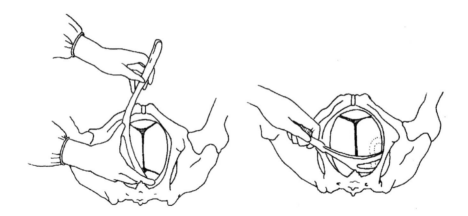

Procedure

1. Insert two fingers of the right hand into the vagina on the side of the fetal

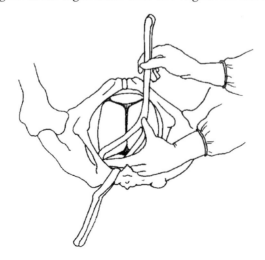

head. Slide the left blade gently between the head and fingers to rest on the side of the head.

2. Repeat the same manoeuvre on the other side, using the left hand and the right blade of the forceps.

3. Depress the handles and lock the forceps.

4. Difficulty in locking usually indicates that the application is incorrect. In this

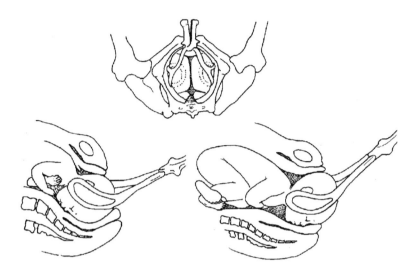

case, remove the blades and recheck position of the head. Reapply only if this is easily possible.

5. After locking, apply steady traction inferiorly and posteriorly with each contraction. Ask the mother to push with each contraction.

6. Between contractions check:
    ○ fetal heart rate
    ○ application of forceps.

7. When the head crowns, make an adequate episiotomy.

[!] **The head should descend with each pull. Only two or three pulls should be necessary.**

8. Perform active management of the third stage of labour to deliver the placenta:
    ○ 10 units oxytocin IM
    ○ controlled cord traction.

9. Check the birth canal for tears following childbirth and repair, if necessary.

10. Repair the episiotomy.

Post-procedure tasks

1. Before removing gloves, dispose of waste materials in a leakproof container or

plastic bag.

2. Use antiseptic hand rub or wash hands thoroughly with soap and water and dry with a clean, dry cloth or air dry.

3. Record the procedure and findings on woman's record.

Failed forceps

■ Classify a failed forceps if:
   ☐ the fetal head does not advance with each pull
   ☐ the fetus is undelivered after three pulls or after 30 minutes.
■ Every application should be considered a trial of forceps. Do not persist if the head does not descend.
■ If forceps delivery fails, perform a **caesarean section**.

[!] **Symphysiotomy is not an option with failed forceps.**

Repair of vaginal and perineal tears

Degrees of tear

There are four degrees of tears that can occur during delivery:

■ First-degree tears involve the vaginal mucosa and connective tissue.
■ Second-degree tears involve the vaginal mucosa, connective tissue and underlying muscles.
■ Third-degree tears involve complete transection of the anal sphincter.
■ Fourth-degree tears involve the rectal mucosa.

Most first-degree tears close spontaneously without sutures.

It is best to suture within the first few hours after the birth. If a tear is not sutured within 12 hours, it is likely to get infected and will not heal as well.

Materials for repair

It is important that absorbable sutures are used for closure. polyglycolic sutures are preferred over chromic catgut for their tensile strength, non-allergenic properties and lower probability of infectious complications.

■ Chromic catgut is an acceptable alternative, but is not ideal.
■ A curved needle for suturing is better than a straight needle.

Pre-procedure tasks

1. Prepare the necessary equipment.

2. Tell the woman (and her support person) what is going to be done, listen to her and respond attentively to her questions and concerns.

3. Provide continual emotional support and reassurance throughout the procedure.

4. Ask about allergies to antiseptics and anaesthetics.

5. Use antiseptic hand rub or wash hands and forearms thoroughly with soap and water and dry with a sterile cloth or air dry.

6. Put on personal protective clothes.

Repair of first- and second-degree tears

1. Ask the woman to position her buttocks toward the lower end of the bed or table (use stirrups if available).

2. Ask an assistant to direct a strong light on to the woman's perineum.

3. Clean the woman's perineum with antiseptic solution.

4. Use local infiltration with lignocaine. If necessary, use a pudendal block.

5. Ask an assistant to massage the uterus and provide fundal pressure.

6. Carefully examine the vagina, perineum and cervix. Use one or two fingers to stretch the vaginal opening to see inside (you might need extra light). Then find the end or tip of the tear. Most tears have only one tip inside, but some have more.

7. It is helpful to gently insert a sterile gauze/tampon in the vagina, above the tear, to reduce the blood flow over the area to be sutured.

[!] **Make sure it is removed when you finish suturing.**

8. If the tear is long and deep through the perineum, inspect to be sure there is no third- or fourth-degree tear:
   ○ place a gloved finger in the anus
   ○ gently lift the finger and identify the sphincter
   ○ feel for the tone or tightness of the sphincter
   ○ change to clean, high-level disinfected gloves.

[!] **If the sphincter is injured, refer to CEOC for repair.**

If the sphincter is not injured, proceed with repair.

9. Apply antiseptic solution to the area around the tear. Make sure there are no known allergies to lignocaine or related drugs.

10. Infiltrate beneath the vaginal mucosa, beneath the skin of the perineum and deeply into the perineal muscle using about 10 ml 0.5% lignocaine solution.

11. Insert the needle along one side of the vaginal incision and inject the lignocaine solution while slowly withdrawing the needle.

12. Repeat on the other side of the vaginal incision and on each side of the perineal incision.

13. Slide the needle under the skin, just inside one of the tears.

14. Slowly inject lignocaine (0.5%) as you slowly pull the needle out.

15. You will see the flesh swell as you inject the lignocaine.

16. Infiltrate the other side of the tear in the same the way.

17. At the conclusion of the set of injections, wait 2 minutes and then pinch the area with forceps. If the woman feels the pinch, wait 2 more minutes and then retest.

[!] **Anaesthetise early to provide sufficient time for effect.**

Repair of vaginal mucosa

Repair the vaginal mucosa using a continuous 2–0 suture:

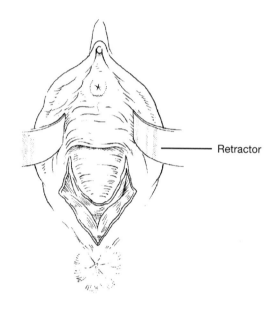

————— Retractor

- Start the repair about 1 cm above the apex (top) of the vaginal tear.
- Continue the suture to the level of the vaginal opening.
- At the opening of the vagina, bring together the cut edges of the vaginal opening.
- Bring the needle under the vaginal opening and out through the perineal tear and tie.

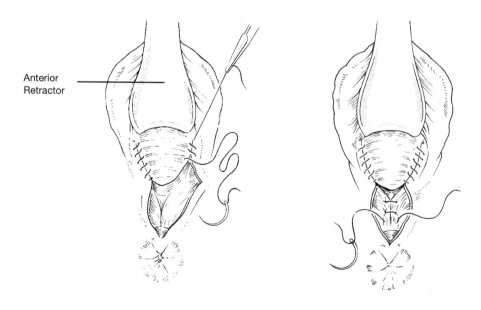

Anterior
Retractor

From time to time, push all the pieces of the tear together to make sure the edges are realigned.

Repair of the perineal muscle layer

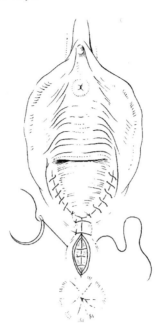

Repair the perineal muscles using interrupted 2-0 suture. If the tear is deep, place a second layer of the same stitch to close the space.

Repair of the skin

Repair the skin using interrupted (or subcuticular) 2-0 sutures starting at the vaginal opening.

Performing a rectal examination

If the tear is deep, perform a rectal examination. Make sure no stitches are in the rectum. If there are, you must take out the sutures and start over again.

Post-procedure
- Place a clean cloth or pad on the woman's perineum.
- Record procedure in woman's notes.

Module 9

Common obstetric emergencies

This module presents four common obstetric emergencies:

■ prolapsed cord
■ shoulder dystocia
■ breech delivery
■ twin delivery.

Aim

■ To recognise when an obstetric emergency (prolapsed cord, shoulder dystocia, breech delivery, twin delivery) has occurred.
■ To practise effective management of the emergencies.

Prolapsed cord

Recognising a prolapsed cord
The umbilical cord is visible at the vagina or is felt on vaginal examination to be coming down, below the presenting part.

Action
■ Check if there are pulsations – feel cord gently.
■ If the cord is pulsating, the fetus is alive.
■ Determine lie of baby and presenting part.

[!] **The baby could be in transverse lie. If the baby is in transverse lie, the mother will need a caesarean section.**

■ If the baby is in longitudinal lie perform a vaginal examination to determine stage of labour.

[!] Your next action will depend upon the findings of vaginal examination.

There are three main options:

1. Cord pulsating: first stage of labour.

2. Cord pulsating: second stage of labour.

3. Cord not pulsating.

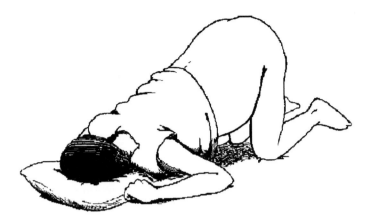

Cord pulsating – first stage of labour (cervix nor fully dilated)

1   Take immediate action to stop presenting part pressing on cord.

There are three possible ways to do this:

1.   Ask the mother to adopt the knee–elbow position (that is, to turn over to face the bed and crouch on all fours raising her buttocks in the air above her shoulders).

[!] The mother can be transferred if necessary in this position.

2.   Manually keep the presenting part out of the pelvis:
   ○ Wearing sterile gloves, insert a hand into the vagina and push the presenting part up to decrease pressure on the cord and dislodge the presenting part from the pelvis.
   ○ Place the other hand on the abdomen in the suprapubic position and keep the presenting part out of the pelvis.
   ○ Once the presenting part is firmly held above the pelvic brim, remove the other hand from the vagina. Keep the hand on the abdomen until the time that the caesarean section is performed.

It is usually only possible to maintain this position for a short time, such as when preparing the mother on the operating table prior to caesarean section or while inserting a catheter.

3.   Fill the bladder:
   ○ Insert a Foley catheter (with balloon), fill the bladder through the catheter with 500–750 ml normal saline then blow up the balloon and clamp the catheter.
   ○ Attach catheter bag as normal but keep catheter clamped and fluid in catheter balloon until baby delivered.
   ○ At caesarean section, release catheter clamp before opening the uterus to empty balloon. Take care not to damage the bladder when opening the abdomen.

This is a very good method of keeping the presenting part away from the prolapsed cord. The woman can easily be transferred in this position.

Once you have taken action to stop the presenting part pressing on the cord:

THEN

Refer to CEOC facility for immediate caesarean section:

- if available, give salbutamol 0.5 mg IV slowly over 2 minutes to reduce contractions
- prepare for resuscitation of the newborn.

Cord pulsating second stage of labour – (cervix fully dilated)
- Expedite delivery with episiotomy and vacuum extraction or forceps.
- If the baby is breech presentation, perform a breech extraction.
- Prepare for resuscitation of the newborn.

Cord not pulsating
- If the cord is not pulsating, the fetus is dead.
- Deliver in the manner that is safest for the woman.

Shoulder dystocia

[!] Be prepared for shoulder dystocia at all deliveries: shoulder dystocia cannot be predicted.

Recognising shoulder dystocia
- The fetal head has been delivered but the shoulders are stuck and cannot be delivered.
- The fetal head is delivered but remains tightly applied to the vulva.
- The chin retracts and depresses the perineum.
- Traction on the head fails to deliver the shoulder, which is caught behind the symphysis pubis.

Action
1. Call for help.

2. Change labour bed to a half-bed or move the woman to lie with her buttocks over the side of the bed.

3. With the woman on her back, ask her to flex both thighs, bringing her knees as far up as possible towards her chest, abduct and rotate legs outwards (McRoberts' position).

[!] Legs should NOT be in lithotomy poles.

4. Apply suprapubic pressure – ask the assistant to use the heel of the hands to push shoulder down and under the symphysis pubis from above.

[!] Do not apply fundal pressure. This will further impact the shoulder and can result in uterine rupture.

5. Make an adequate episiotomy to reduce soft tissue obstruction and to allow space for manipulation.

6. Apply firm, continuous traction downwards on the fetal head to move the shoulder that is anterior under the symphysis pubis.

[!] **Avoid excessive traction on the head as this may result in brachial plexus injury.**

7. If the shoulder still is not delivered:
    ○ insert a hand into the vagina along the baby's back
    ○ apply pressure to the anterior shoulder in the direction of the baby's chest (sternum) to rotate the shoulder and decrease the shoulder diameter
    ○ if needed, apply pressure to the shoulder that is posterior in the direction of the sternum.

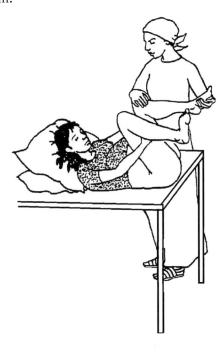

8. If the shoulder still is not delivered despite the above measures, try to deliver the posterior shoulder first:
    ○ grasp the humerus of the arm that is posterior and, keeping the arm flexed at the elbow, sweep the arm across the chest. This will provide room for the shoulder that is anterior to move under the symphysis pubis.

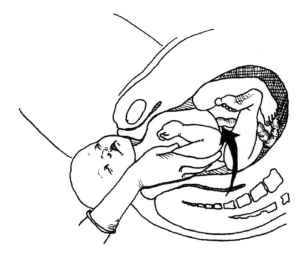

9. If all of the above measures fail to deliver the shoulder, other options include:
    ○ turning the woman on all fours (knee–elbow position) and repeating all the previous measures
    ○ fracturing the clavicle to decrease the width of the shoulders and freeing the shoulder that is anterior
    ○ applying traction with a hook in the axilla to extract the arm that is posterior.

10. When the baby is delivered, wipe baby dry, wrap in warm cloth and put in skin-to-skin contact with the mother.

11. Perform active management of the third stage of labour to deliver the placenta:
    ○ 10 units oxytocin IM
    ○ controlled cord traction.

12. Check the birth canal for tears following childbirth and repair episiotomy.

Post-procedure tasks
1. Before removing gloves, dispose of waste materials in a leakproof container or plastic bag.

2. Use antiseptic hand rub or wash hands thoroughly with soap and water and dry with a clean, dry cloth or air dry.

3. Record the procedure and findings on the woman's record.

4. Explain what happened to the woman and her support person.

Breech delivery

Recognising a breech presentation
A breech presentation may be discovered during abdominal palpation and/or may be confirmed by vaginal examination during labour.

Conditions necessary for breech delivery
■ Complete or frank breech.
■ Adequate clinical pelvimetry, especially that sacral promontory is not tipped.
■ Fetus is not too large.
■ No previous caesarean section for cephalopelvic disproportion.

Preparation for a breech delivery
1. Prepare the necessary equipment for delivery and resuscitation of the newborn.

2. Tell the woman (and her support person) what is going to be done, listen to her and respond attentively to her questions and concerns.

3. Provide continual emotional support and reassurance.

5. Start an IV infusion.

6.   If necessary, use a pudendal block.

7.   Ensure that the cervix is fully dilated and that contractions are regular and strong.

Pre-procedure tasks

1.   Use antiseptic hand rub or wash hands thoroughly with soap and water and dry with a sterile cloth or air dry and put on sterile gloves.

2.   Clean the vulva with antiseptic solution.

3.   Drape the mother.

4.   Catheterize the bladder, if necessary.

Procedure
Delivery of the buttocks and legs

1.   Allow delivery to proceed without any interference until the buttocks are visible.

2.   As the buttocks enter the vagina and are visible: **WATCH.**

3.   As the perineum distends, decide whether an episiotomy is necessary. If needed, provide perineal infiltration with lignocaine and perform an episiotomy.

4.   Let the buttocks deliver until the shoulder blades (scapulae) are seen.

[!] **DO NOT PULL OR INTERFERE IN ANY WAY.**

5.   Gently hold the buttocks in one hand, but do not pull.

6.   If the legs do not deliver spontaneously, deliver one leg at a time:
     ○ push behind the knee to bend the leg
     ○ grasp the ankle and deliver the foot and leg
     ○ repeat for the other leg.

7.   Hold the newborn by the hips, but do not pull.

8.   Ask the mother to continue pushing with contractions.

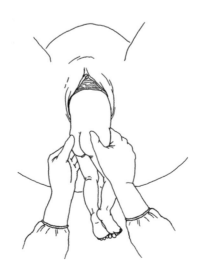

Delivery of the arms

9. If the arms are felt on the chest, allow them to disengage spontaneously (that is, without interference), one by one:

    ○ after spontaneous delivery of the first arm, lift the buttocks toward the mother's abdomen to enable the second arm to deliver spontaneously

    ○ if the arm does not deliver spontaneously, place one or two fingers in the elbow and bend the arm, bringing the hand down over the newborn's face.

10. If the arms are stretched above the head or folded around the neck, use Lovset's manoeuvre:

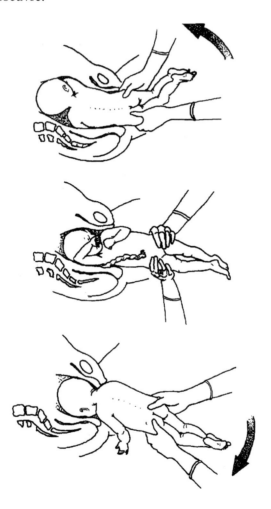

Lovset's manoeuvre

■ Hold the newborn by the hips and turn half a circle, keeping the back uppermost.

■ Apply downward traction at the same time so that the posterior arm becomes anterior and deliver the arm under the pubic arch by placing one or two fingers on the upper part of the arm.

■ Draw the arm down over the chest as the elbow is flexed, with the hand sweeping over the face.

■ To deliver the second arm, turn the newborn back half a circle while keeping the back uppermost and applying downward traction to deliver the second arm in the same way under the pubic arch.

11. If the newborn's body cannot be turned to deliver the arm that is anterior
    first, deliver the arm that is posterior:
    ○ hold and lift the newborn up by the ankles
    ○ move the newborn's chest toward the woman's inner leg to deliver the
       posterior shoulder
    ○ deliver the arm and hand
    ○ move the baby down by the ankles to deliver the anterior shoulder
    ○ deliver the arm and hand.

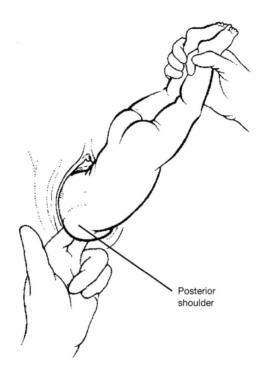

Posterior
shoulder

Delivery of the head

12. After the arms are delivered, allow the head to descend until the hairline is
    visible then deliver the head by the Mauriceau-Smellie-Veit manoeuvre:
    ○ Lay baby face down with the length of its body over your hand and arm.
    ○ Place first and third fingers of this hand on the baby's cheekbones.
    ○ Use the other hand to grasp the newborn's shoulders.
    ○ With two fingers of this hand, gently flex the baby's head toward the chest
       to encourage flexion of the head.
    ○ At the same time apply downward pressure on the jaw to bring the baby's
       head down.
    ○ Pull gently to deliver the head.
    ○ Ask an assistant to push gently above the mother's pubic bone as the head
       delivers.
    ○ Raise the baby (still astride the arm) until the mouth and nose are free.

13. As soon as the baby is delivered, wipe dry, wrap in a warm cloth and put in
    skin-to-skin contact with the mother.

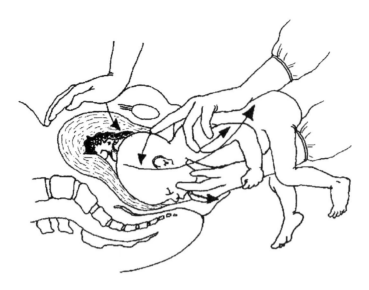

Entrapped (stuck) head

Apply firm pressure above the mother's pubic bone to flex the baby's head and push it through the pelvis. If available, you can use forceps to try to deliver the head:

■ Wrap the baby's body in a cloth or towel and hold the baby up. Ask an assistant to hold the baby while you apply the forceps blades.
■ Place the left blade of the forceps over the baby's head as for forceps delivery working under the body of the baby.
■ Place the right blade and lock handles.
■ Use the forceps to flex and deliver the baby's head.

After delivery:

14. Perform active management of the third stage of labour to deliver the placenta:
    ○ 10 units oxytocin IM
    ○ controlled cord traction.

15. Check the birth canal for tears following childbirth and repair episiotomy if necessary.

Post-procedure tasks

1. Before removing gloves, dispose of waste materials in a leakproof container or plastic bag.

2 Use antiseptic hand rub or wash hands thoroughly with soap and water and dry with a clean, dry cloth or air dry.

3. Record the procedure and findings on woman's record.

4. Explain what happened to the woman and her support person

Footling breech

A footling breech should usually be delivered by caesarean section unless:

■ advanced labour with fully dilated cervix and referral for caesarean section not possible before birth
■ preterm baby that is not likely to survive after delivery
■ you are delivering a second baby (for example in twins or triplets).

To deliver the baby vaginally

1. Grasp the baby's ankles with one hand.

2. If only one foot presents, insert a hand into the vagina and gently pull the baby downwards by the ankles.

3. Deliver the baby until the back and shoulder blades are seen.

4. Proceed with the delivery of the arms.

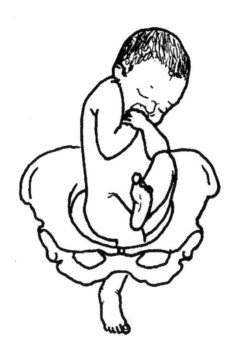

Breech extraction

■ Wearing sterile gloves, insert a hand into the uterus and grasp the baby's foot.
■ Exert traction on the foot until the buttocks are seen.
■ Proceed with delivery of the arms.
■ Give a single dose of prophylactic antibiotics after breech extraction:
  ☐ ampicillin 2 g IV PLUS metronidazole 500 mg IV

  OR

  ☐ cefazolin 1 g IV PLUS metronidazole 500 mg IV.

Twin delivery

Recognising a twin presentation

A twin presentation may be discovered by abdominal palpation, confirmed by ultra sound scan or by abdominal palpation and/or vaginal examination after delivery of first baby.

Preparation

1. Prepare the necessary equipment for delivery and resuscitation of two babies.

2. Tell the woman (and her support person) what is going to be done, listen to her and respond attentively to her questions and concerns.

3. Provide continual emotional support and reassurance.

4. Monitor fetuses by intermittent auscultation of the fetal heart rates.

5. Monitor progress in labour using a partograph.

First baby

1. Start an IV infusion. Prepare in case oxytocin infusion will be needed after the first twin is delivered.

2. Check presentation of first baby:
   ○ if a vertex presentation, allow labour to progress as for a single vertex presentation
   ○ if a breech presentation, apply the same guidelines as for a singleton breech presentation
   ○ if a transverse lie, deliver by caesarean section.

[!] Leave a clamp on the maternal end of the umbilical cord and do not attempt to deliver the placenta until the last baby is delivered.

Second baby

3. Immediately after the first baby is delivered, perform a vaginal examination to determine:
   ○ if the cord has prolapsed
   ○ whether the membranes are intact or ruptured
   ○ presentation of other baby: vertex or breech, transverse lie.

4. Palpate the abdomen to determine lie of second baby.

5. Correct to longitudinal lie, manually if necessary if possible.

6. Check fetal heart rate.

Vertex presentation:

■ If the fetal head is not engaged, encourage longitudinal lie and head descent into the pelvis manually (hands on the abdomen).
■ If the membranes are intact, carry out **controlled** rupture of the membranes and facilitate descent of the head into the pelvis.
■ Continue to check fetal heart rate between contractions.

- If contractions are inadequate after the birth of the first baby, augment labour with oxytocin using a rapid escalation to produce good contractions (three contractions in 10 minutes, each lasting more than 40 seconds).
- If spontaneous delivery does not occur within 2 hours of good contractions or if there are fetal heart rate abnormalities (less than 100 beats/minute or more than 180 beats/minute), deliver by assisted delivery (vacuum extraction) or caesarean section.

Breech presentation:

- If the baby is estimated to be no larger than the first baby, and if the cervix has not contracted, prepare for breech delivery.
- If there are inadequate or no contractions after the birth of the first baby, escalate oxytocin infusion at a rapid but controlled rate to produce good contractions (three contractions in 10 minutes, each lasting more than 40 seconds).
- If the membranes, are intact, rupture them once the breech has descended.
- Check fetal heart rate between contractions. If there are fetal heart rate abnormalities (less than 100 beats/minutes or more than 180 beats/minute), deliver by breech extraction.
- If vaginal delivery is not possible, deliver by caesarean section.

Non-longitudinal presentation:

- Correct the lie of the baby to longitudinal by external cephalic version if possible.
- If external cephalic version is not possible, attempt internal podalic version if a foot is palpable vaginally and membranes are intact (or only just ruptured):
  - ☐ Grasp a foot and exert gentle, steady traction between contractions.
  - ☐ Rupture the membranes when the lie is longitudinal and breech is in the vagina.
  - ☐ Deliver as singleton breech.
- If the lie does not become longitudinal with gentle, steady traction, deliver by caesarean section.

- Check the birth canal for tears following childbirth and repair episiotomy, if one was performed.

Post-procedure tasks

1. Before removing gloves, dispose of waste materials in a leakproof container or plastic bag.

2. Use antiseptic hand rub or wash hands thoroughly with soap and water and dry with a clean, dry cloth or air dry.

3. Record the procedure and findings on woman's record.

4. Explain what happened to the mother and her support person.

Module 10

Complications of abortion

Aim

- ■ To recognise the presentation of complications of abortion.
- ■ To practise effective management of the complications of abortion, including the use of manual vacuum aspiration.

Recognising complications of abortion

Diagnosis and management of complications of abortion

Symptoms and signs	Complications	Management
Lower abdominal pain Rebound tenderness Tender uterus Prolonged bleeding Malaise Fever Foul-smelling vaginal discharge Purulent cervical discharge Cervical motion tenderness	Infection/sepsis	Begin antibiotics as soon as possible before attempting manual vacuum aspiration
Cramping/abdominal pain Rebound tenderness Abdominal distension Rigid (tense and hard) abdomen Shoulder pain Nausea/vomiting Fever	Uterine, vaginal or bowel injuries	Perform a laparotomy to repair the injury and perform manual vacuum aspiration simultaneously. Seek further assistance if required

Initial assessment

1. Greet the woman respectfully and with kindness.

2. Assess patient for shock and sepsis (see **Modules 2 and 7**).

Medical evaluation

1. Take a history and perform physical (heart, lungs and abdomen) and pelvic examinations.

2. Perform laboratory tests if possible: haemoglobin, thick slide for malaria parasites, urine microscopy and dipstick.

3. Give the woman information about her condition and what to expect.

4. Discuss her need for family planning.

Manual vacuum aspiration (MVA)

Preparation

1. Tell the woman (and her support person) what is going to be done, listen to her and respond attentively to her questions and concerns. Provide continual emotional support and reassurance.

2. Tell her that she may feel discomfort during some of the steps of the procedure and you will tell her in advance when this is likely to happen.

3. Give paracetamol 500 mg by mouth to the woman 30 minutes before the procedure.

4. Ask about allergies to antiseptics and anaesthetics.

5. Determine that the necessary equipment and supplies are present:
   ○ make sure that the required sterile instruments are present
   ○ make sure that the appropriate sizes of cannula and adapters are available.

6. Check the MVA syringe and charge it (establish vacuum). Assemble the syringe; close the pinch valve; pull back on the plunger until the plunger arms lock.

[!] **For molar pregnancy, when the uterine contents are likely to be copious, have three syringes ready for use.**

7. Check that the woman has recently emptied her bladder.

8. Check that she has thoroughly washed and rinsed her perineal area.

9. Wash hands thoroughly with soap and water and dry with a sterile cloth or air dry. Put on personal protective equipment and gloves.

Pre-procedure tasks

1. Inform the woman of each step in the procedure prior to performing it.

2. Give oxytocin 10 units IM or ergometrine 0.2 mg IM before the procedure to make the myometrium firmer and reduce the risk of perforation.

3. Perform bimanual pelvic examination, checking the size and position of uterus and degree of cervical dilatation.

4. Give paracervical block.

5. Prepare 20 ml 0.5% lignocaine solution without adrenaline.

6. Draw 10 ml 0.5% lignocaine solution into a syringe.

7. If using a single-toothed tenaculum, inject 1 ml lignocaine solution into the anterior or posterior lip of the cervix (the 10 o'clock or 12 o'clock position is usually used).

8. Gently grasp anterior or posterior lip of the cervix with a single-toothed tenaculum or vulsella forceps (preferably, use ring or sponge forceps if incomplete abortion).

9. With tenaculum or vulsella forceps on the cervix, use slight traction and movement to help identify the area between the smooth cervical epithelium and the vaginal tissue.

10. Insert the needle just under the epithelium and aspirate by drawing the plunger back slightly to make sure the needle is not penetrating a blood vessel.

11. Inject about 2 ml 0.5% lignocaine solution just under the epithelium, not deeper than 3 mm, at 3, 5, 7 and 9 o'clock.

12. Wait 2 minutes and then pinch the cervix with the forceps (f the patient feels the pinch, wait 2 more minutes and then retest).

Procedure

1. Insert the speculum and remove blood or tissue from vagina using sponge forceps and gauze.

2. Apply antiseptic solution to cervix and vagina three times using gauze or cotton sponge.

3. Remove any products of conception from the cervical os and check cervix for tears.

[!] **With incomplete abortion, a ring or sponge forceps is preferable, as it is less likely than the tenaculum to tear the cervix with traction and does not require the use of lignocaine for placement.**

4. Gently apply traction on the cervix to straighten the cervical canal and uterine cavity.

5. If necessary, dilate the cervix using progressively larger cannula.

[!] **Dilatation is needed only in cases of missed abortion or when products of conception have remained in the uterus for several days.**

6. Insert the cannula. Slowly push the cannula into the uterine cavity until it touches the fundus, but not more than 10 cm. Measure the depth of the uterus by dots visible on the cannula and then withdraw the cannula slightly.

7. Attach the prepared MVA syringe to the cannula by holding the vulsella (or tenaculum) and the end of the cannula in one hand and the syringe in the

other. Release the pinch valve(s) on the syringe to transfer the vacuum through the cannula to the uterine cavity.

8. Evacuate remaining contents by gently rotating the syringe from side to side (10 to 12 o'clock) and then moving the cannula gently and slowly back and forth within the uterine cavity.

[!] **To avoid losing the vacuum, do not withdraw the cannula opening past the cervical os. If the vacuum is lost or if the syringe is more than half full, empty it and then re-establish the vacuum.**

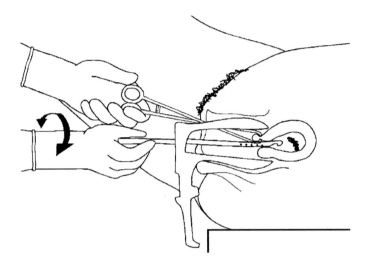

9. Evacuate any remaining contents of the uterine cavity by rotating the cannula and syringe from 10 o'clock to 2 o'clock and moving the cannula gently and slowly back and forth within the uterus:
   ○ If the syringe becomes half full before the procedure is complete, detach the cannula from the syringe. Remove only the syringe, leaving the cannula in place.
   ○ Push the plunger to empty the contents into the strainer.
   ○ Recharge syringe, attach to cannula and release pinch valve(s).
   ○ Check for signs of completion (red or pink foam, no more tissue in cannula, a 'gritty' sensation and uterus contracts around the cannula). Withdraw the cannula and MVA syringe gently.

[!] Avoid grasping the syringe by the plunger arms while the vacuum is established and the cannula is in the uterus. If the plunger arms become unlocked, the plunger may accidentally slip back into the syringe, pushing material back into the uterus.

10. Remove cannula from the MVA syringe and push the plunger to empty contents into the strainer.

[!] **Place the empty syringe on a high-level disinfected tray or container until you are certain the procedure is complete.**

11. Remove tenaculum or forceps from the cervix before removing the speculum.

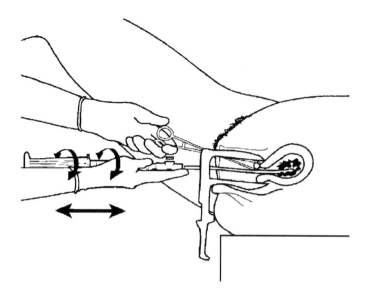

12. Perform bimanual examination to check size and firmness of uterus.

13. Rinse the tissue with water or saline, if necessary.

14. Quickly inspect the tissue removed from the uterus to be sure the uterus is completely evacuated.

15. If no products of conception are seen:
    ○ All of the products of conception may have been passed before the MVA was performed (complete abortion).
    ○ The uterine cavity may appear to be empty but may not have been emptied completely. Repeat the evacuation.
    ○ The vaginal bleeding may not have been caused by an incomplete abortion (for instance, it may have been breakthrough bleeding, as may be seen with hormonal contraceptives or uterine fibroids).
    ○ The uterus may be abnormal (that is, the cannula may have been inserted in the non-pregnant side of a double uterus).

[!] **Absence of products of conception in a woman with symptoms of pregnancy raises the strong possibility of ectopic pregnancy.**

16. Gently insert a speculum into the vagina and examine for bleeding. If the uterus is still soft and not smaller or if there is persistent, brisk bleeding, repeat the evacuation.

Post-procedure tasks

1. Before removing gloves, dispose of waste materials in a leakproof container or plastic bag.

2. Place all instruments in 0.5% chlorine solution for 10 minutes for decontamination.

3. Dispose of needle or syringe, flush needles and syringes with 0.5% chlorine solution three times, then place in a puncture-proof container.

4. Attach used cannula to MVA syringe and flush both with 0.5% chlorine solution.

5. Detach cannula from syringe and soak them in 0.5% chlorine solution for 10 minutes for decontamination.

6. Empty products of conception and dispose of these in a respectful and safe manner.

7. Wash hands thoroughly with soap and water and dry with a clean, dry cloth or air dry.

8. Allow the patient to rest comfortably for at least 60 minutes, where her recovery can be monitored.

9. Check for bleeding and ensure that cramping has decreased before discharge.

10. Instruct patient regarding post-abortion care and warning signs:
    ○ prolonged cramping (more than a few days)
    ○ prolonged bleeding (more than 2 weeks)
    ○ bleeding more than normal menstrual bleeding
    ○ severe or increased pain
    ○ fever, chills or malaise
    ○ fainting.

11. Tell her when to return if follow up is needed and that she can return anytime she has concerns.

12. Encourage the woman to eat, drink and walk about as she wishes.

13. Discuss reproductive goals and, as appropriate, provide family planning.

14. Discharge women with uncomplicated cases in 1–2 hours.

Appendix 1.
Supporting normal birth

Key points for good care during normal labour and delivery

- Presence of a birth partner or companion. Supportive care during labour is the most important thing to help the woman tolerate labour pains and facilitate the progress of labour.
- Privacy ensured.
- Good communication and building trust with staff.
- Encourage walking around and changing positions frequently.
- Encourage adequate intake of food and drinks.
- Monitor maternal and fetal wellbeing using the partograph.
- Allow the women to adopt her position of choice for delivery; for example, squatting, lying down, on all fours, upright.

Care that is of no benefit and should be abandoned

- Routine shaving of the pudendal area.
- Giving an enema.
- Routinely cutting an episiotomy for delivery.

Normal labour and delivery

Progress in first stage of labour
Findings suggestive of satisfactory progress in first stage of labour are:

- Regular contractions of progressively increasing frequency and duration to three contractions in 10 minutes each lasting 40 seconds or more.
- Rate of cervical dilatation at least 1 cm/hour during the active phase of labour (cervical dilatation on or to the left of alert line of the partograph).
- Cervix well applied to the presenting part.

Progress in second stage of labour
Findings suggestive of satisfactory progress in second stage of labour are:

- Steady descent of fetus through birth canal.
- Onset of expulsive (pushing) phase.

Once the cervix is fully dilated and the woman is in the expulsive phase of the second stage, encourage the woman to assume the position she prefers and encourage her to push.

Delivery of the head

- Ask the woman to pant or give only small pushes with contractions as the baby's head delivers.
- To control birth of the head, place the fingers of one hand against the baby's head to keep it flexed (bent).
- Continue to gently support the perineum as the baby's head delivers.
- Once the baby's head delivers, ask the woman not to push.
- Feel around the baby's neck for the umbilical cord:
  - ☐ if the cord is around the neck but is loose, slip it over the baby's head
  - ☐ if the cord is tight around the neck, doubly clamp and cut it before unwinding it from around the neck.

Completion of delivery

- Allow the baby's head to turn spontaneously.
- After the head turns, place a hand on each side of the baby's head. Tell the woman to push gently with the next contraction.
- Reduce tears by delivering one shoulder at a time. Move the baby's head posteriorly to deliver the shoulder that is anterior.
- Lift the baby's head anteriorly to deliver the shoulder that is posterior.
- Support the rest of the baby's body with one hand as it slides out.
- Clamp and cut the umbilical cord.

[!] Most babies begin crying or breathing spontaneously within 30 seconds of birth.

- Place the baby on the mother's abdomen or chest. Thoroughly dry the baby, wipe the eyes and assess the baby's breathing.
- Ensure that the baby is kept warm and in skin-to-skin contact on the mother's chest. Wrap the baby in a soft, dry cloth, cover with a blanket and ensure the head is covered to prevent heat loss.
- Palpate the abdomen to rule out the presence of an additional baby(s) and proceed with active management of the third stage.

Active management of the third stage

Active management of the third stage helps prevent postpartum haemorrhage. Active management of the third stage of labour includes:

- early clamping and division of the umbilical cord
- prophylactic use of oxytocin (see below)
- controlled cord traction for delivery of the placenta.

Prophylactic oxytocin to prevent postpartum haemorrhage

■ Within 1 minute of delivery of the baby, palpate the abdomen to rule out the presence of an additional baby(s) and give oxytocin 10 units IM.

■ Oxytocin is preferred because it is effective 2–3 minutes after injection, has minimal adverse effects and can be used in all women. If oxytocin is not available, give ergometrine 0.2 mg IM or prostaglandins. Make sure there is no additional baby(s) before giving these medications.

[!] **Do not give ergometrine to women with pre-eclampsia, eclampsia or high blood pressure because it may increase the blood pressure and risk of cerebrovascular accidents.**

Controlled cord traction

■ Clamp the cord close to the perineum using sponge forceps. Hold the clamped cord and the end of forceps with one hand.

■ Place the other hand just above the woman's pubic bone and stabilise the uterus by applying counter traction during controlled cord traction. This helps prevent inversion of the uterus.

■ Keep slight tension on the cord and await a strong uterine contraction (2–3 minutes).

■ When the uterus becomes rounded or the cord lengthens, very gently pull downward on the cord to deliver the placenta. Do not wait for a gush of blood before applying traction on the cord. Continue to apply counter traction to the uterus with the other hand.

■ If the placenta does not descend during 30–40 seconds of controlled cord traction (that is, there are no signs of placental separation), do not continue to pull on the cord.

■ Gently hold the cord and wait until the uterus is well contracted again. If necessary, use a sponge forceps to clamp the cord closer to the perineum as it lengthens.

■ With the next contraction, repeat controlled cord traction with counter traction.

[!] **Never apply cord traction (pull) without applying counter traction (push) above the pubic bone with the other hand.**

[!] **Note that using fundal pressure can lead to inversion of the uterus.**

[!] **Routinely 'rubbing up a contraction' is not good practice. This should only be done in case of postpartum haemorrhage (Module 5).**

■ As the placenta delivers, the thin membranes can tear off. Hold the placenta in two hands and gently turn it until the membranes are twisted.

■ Slowly pull to complete the delivery.

■ If the membranes tear, gently examine the upper vagina and cervix wearing high-level disinfected gloves and use a sponge forceps to remove any pieces of membrane that are present.

■ Look carefully at the placenta to be sure none of it is missing. If a portion of the maternal surface is missing or there are torn membranes with vessels, suspect retained placental fragments.

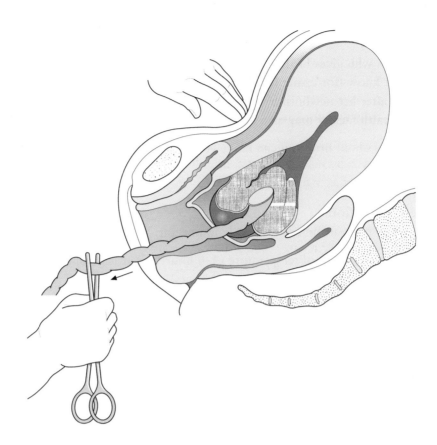

Examination for tears
- ■ Examine the woman carefully and repair any tears to the cervix or vagina or repair the episiotomy.
- ■ Explain all procedures to the mother and her support person.

Initial care of the newborn

- ■ Check the baby's breathing and colour every 5 minutes.
- ■ Check warmth by feeling the baby's feet every 15 minutes:
  - ☐ if the baby's feet feel cold, check axillary temperature
  - ☐ if the baby's temperature is below 36.5°C, re-warm the baby.
- ■ Check the cord for bleeding every 15 minutes. If the cord is bleeding, retie cord more tightly.
- ■ Wipe off any meconium or blood from skin.
- ■ Encourage breastfeeding when the baby appears ready (begins 'rooting'). Do not force the baby to the breast.

Avoid separating mother from baby whenever possible. Do not leave mother and baby unattended at any time.

Postpartum care for the woman

A new mother needs both emotional support and practical help.

[!] **A woman who gives birth in unfamiliar surroundings attended by people she does not know (for example, in a health facility) may feel inhibited and unable to look after her newborn baby as she would do at home. Rules and policies in the health facility may also obstruct immediate postnatal social interaction.**

Think carefully about how you can make your facility more client friendly in this respect!

Routine observations

The first hours postpartum are extremely important:

- Regular measurement of temperature (4–6 hourly or at least once before discharge if women discharged within 8 hours).
- Regular measurement of BP and pulse (4–6 hourly).
- Regular check for vaginal loss (4–6 hourly).
- Regular check of fundal height (4–6 hourly).
- Pain relief: pain in perineum and breasts is common and women often count these as unpleasant memories of childbirth. Give simple regular pain relief medication, such as paracetamol.

Identify any signs of serious maternal complications, in particular haemorrhage, eclampsia and infections. Start treatment immediately if any of these occur; see Modules on haemorrhage (Module 5), eclampsia (Module 4) and sepsis (Module 7).

Length of stay in health facility

- A healthy mother and baby do not need to stay at the facility except by their own choice, for instance if their home is far away and there is no supportive care at home.
- A healthy mother and baby who have help at home, have been informed of and understand danger signs that should prompt them to seek health care and who wish to go home may be discharged safely within 6–48 hours from birth.
- Decisions on when a woman should go home after childbirth should always be based on the mother's individual needs and preferences rather than on a predetermined formula.

Appendix 2
Partograph

Starting the partograph

A partograph chart must only be started when a woman is in established labour, also known as the active phase of labour.

The latent phase (slow period of cervical dilatation) is from 0 cm to 3 cm with a gradual shortening of the cervix.

The active phase (faster period of cervical dilatation) is from 3 cm to 10 cm (full cervical dilatation).

In the active phase, contractions must be three or more in 10 minutes, each lasting 40 seconds or more.

Using the partograph

The WHO partograph has been modified to make it simpler and easier to use. The latent phase has been removed and plotting on the partograph begins in the active phase when the cervix is 3–4 cm dilated. Note that the partograph should be enlarged to full size before use. Record the following on the partograph:

- **Patient information:** Fill out name, gravida, para, hospital number, date and time of admission and time of ruptured membranes.
- **Fetal heart rate:** record every half hour.
- The first entry on the partograph is made on the '0' hours timeline and subsequent entries are related to that line.
- **Amniotic fluid:** record the colour of amniotic fluid at every vaginal examination:
  - ☐ **I:** membranes intact
  - ☐ **C:** membranes ruptured, clear fluid
  - ☐ **M:** meconium-stained fluid
  - ☐ **B:** blood-stained fluid.

- **Moulding:**
  - ☐ 1: sutures apposed
  - ☐ 2: sutures overlapped but reducible
  - ☐ 3: sutures overlapped and not reducible.

- **Cervical dilatation:** assessed at every vaginal examination and marked with a cross (**X**). Begin plotting on the partograph at 4 cm.

- **Alert line:** a line starts at 3–4 cm of cervical dilatation to the point of expected full dilatation at the rate of 1 cm/hour.

■ **Action line:** parallel and 4 hours to the right of the alert line.

■ **Descent assessed by abdominal palpation:** refers to the part of the head (divided

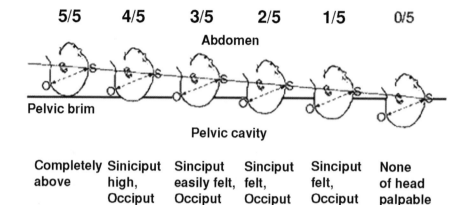

5/5	4/5	3/5	2/5	1/5	0/5
Completely above	Siniciput high, Occiput easily felt	Sinciput easily felt, Occiput felt	Sinciput felt, Occiput just felt	Sinciput felt, Occiput not felt	None of head palpable

into five parts) palpable above the symphysis pubis; recorded as a circle (O) at every vaginal examination. At 0/5, the sinciput (S) is at the level of the symphysis pubis.

■ **Hours:** refers to the time elapsed since onset of active phase of labour (observed or extrapolated).

■ **Time:** record actual time.

■ **Contractions:** chart every half hour; palpate the number of contractions in 10 minutes and their duration in seconds.

   ☐ less than 20 seconds:

   ☐ between 20 and 40 seconds:

   ☐ more than 40 seconds:

■ **Oxytocin:** record the amount of oxytocin/volume intravenous fluids in drops/minute every 30 minutes when used.

■ **Drugs given:** record any additional drugs given.

■ **Pulse:** record every 30 minutes and mark with a dot (.).

■ **Blood pressure:** record every 4 hours and mark with arrows.

■ **Temperature:** record every 2 hours.

■ **Protein, acetone and volume:** record every time urine is passed.

The modified WHO Partograph

Name _____   Gravida _____   Para _____   Hospital number _____

Date of admission _____   Time of admission _____   Ruptured membranes _____   hours

Fetal heart rate (200, 190, 180, 170, 160, 150, 140, 130, 120, 110, 100, 90, 80)

Amniotic fluid
Moulding

Cervix (cm) [Plot X] (10, 9, 8, 7, 6, 5, 4, 3, 2, 1, 0)

Alert   Action

Descent of head [Plot O]

Hours

Time

Contractions per 10 mins (5, 4, 3, 2, 1)

Oxytocin U/L drops/min

Drugs given and IV fluids

Pulse ● and BP (180, 170, 160, 150, 140, 130, 120, 110, 100, 90, 80, 70, 60)

Temp °C

Urine { protein, acetone, volume }

Illustration of position of fetal head

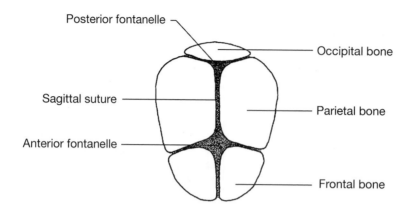

Posterior fontanelle — | — Occipital bone
Sagittal suture — | — Parietal bone
Anterior fontanelle — | — Frontal bone

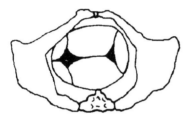

Left occiput transverse

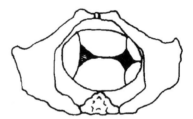

Right occiput transverse

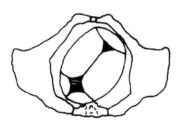

Left occiput anterior

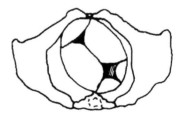

Right occiput anterior

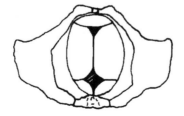

Occiput anterior

Appendix 3

Essential drugs and immunisations with dosage and estimated need for pregnancy, childbirth and newborn care

Drug[1]	Dosage	Estimated amounts needed/1000 deliveries[2]	Notes
1. Drugs for resuscitation			
Adrenaline (epinephrine)	Adult CPR: 1mg IV every 3 minutes Adult anaphylactic shock: 1.0 mg IM every 10 minutes or 50–100 microgram IV Neonatal resuscitation: 10 micrograms/kilo IV (= 25–30 micrograms for average small baby)	Comes in vials 1/10,000 (100 micrograms/ml) in 10-ml ampoules **Suggest 5 ampoules**	For emergency box only
Atropine sulphate	Adult CPR: 3 mg as single dose Give 0.3–0.6 mg if heart rate < 45 beats/minute	1-ml ampoules of 600 micrograms/ml **Suggest 5 ampoules** (of 1 ml 600 micrograms/ml) **Note:** other strengths also available: pre-filled disposable syringe atropine sulphate 100 micrograms/ml pre-filled disposable syringe atropine sulphate 200 micrograms/ml Both available in 5-ml and 10-ml syringes	For emergency box only **Note**: atropine not used in neonatal resuscitation
Dextrose (or glucose)	Neonatal resuscitation: bolus of 5 ml/kg of 10% **Note**: for neonates, 50% solution needed, which can be diluted to 10% OR provide 10% dextrose/glucose 5% dextrose may be useful in the treatment of cerebral malaria	5% or 50% can be used and diluted if needed **Estimated need: 10 vials in total of 5% and/or 50% dextrose/glucose**	For emergency box only

Drug[1]	Dosage	Estimated amounts needed/1000 deliveries[2]	Notes
Ephedrine hydrochloride	**For reversal of spinal anaesthesia** (if BP falls by more than 20%) Give by slow iv injection: 3 mg increments every 3–4 minutes according to response BP to maximum 30 mg Ephedrine hydrochloride 3mg/ml in 10 ml ampoules	**Estimated need: 10 ampoules of 10 ml ephedrine hydrochloride**	For emergency box only

2. Antibiotics

Amoxicillin	500mg capsules for oral use	Oral dose; up to 500 mg 8-hourly 7 days' treatment = 21 capsules of 500 mg/full course **Estimated need: 15% = 150 cases = 3150 capsules of 500 mg for oral use**	Better absorbed than ampicillin when given orally – amoxicillin preferred in pregnancy if oral antibiotic needed
Ampicillin	500 mg powder (ampoules) for reconstitution for IV use	Estimate average regimen at: IV dose 1 g start then 500 mg 6-hourly for 5 days (can move to oral) = 22 doses of 500 mg IV/case **Estimated need: 5% = 50 cases = 1100 ampoules of 500 mg for IV use**	**For neonatal sepsis[3]** use ampicillin IV (covers *Listeria*) or penicillin IV plus gentamycin **Neonatal dose**: 25 mg/kg ampicillin or penicillin and gentamycin (age up to 2 weeks: 3 mg/kg 12-hourly; age 2 weeks to 12 years: 2 mg/kg 8-hourly)
Benzylpenicillin (penicillin G)	1-g vial of powder for injection (or 3-g vial) OR benzathine benzylpenicillin powder for injection 1.44 g benzyl penicillin (= 2.4 million units) in 5-ml vial[4] Often given stat 2.4 million units IM	Assuming 5% incidence antenatal syphilis = 100 treatment doses needed (woman AND partner)[5] **Estimated need: 100 vials 5 ml benzyl penicillin**	

Drug[1]	Dosage	Estimated amounts needed/1000 deliveries[2]	Notes
Cephalosporin[6] (e.g. cefazolin, cefotaxime, ceftriaxone)	Dosage will be 500 mg either IV or oral (but in some cases 1 g)	Assuming 5% incidence life-threatening complications, including sepsis, requiring cephalosporin: Estimate average IV regimen at 500 mg 8-hourly for 5 days (can then move to oral) = 15 doses/case **Estimate 50 cases = 750 doses of 500 mg IV cephalosporin (ampoules)** Estimate similar amount for oral use: **750 doses 500 mg cephalosporin for oral use (capsules)**	Generally to use as second (not first) choice antibiotic in cases of severe sepsis. Mostly IV will be needed to commence but may need to be continued orally to complete dose
Erythromycin	500 mg capsules for oral use	Common regimen: 500 mg 6-hourly for 7 days = 28 capsules/case **Estimated need: 5% of cases = 50 cases = 1400 doses of 500 mg for oral use (capsules)**	Could be used instead of penicillin where penicillin sensitivity, otherwise not often used.

Drug[1]	Dosage	Estimated amounts needed/1000 deliveries[2]	Notes
Gentamicin (aminoglycoside)	A common dose in adults is 80 mg; use 2-ml vials for reconstitution with 40 mg/ml (i.e. each 2-ml vial = 1 dose)	Assuming 5% incidence life-threatening complications, including sepsis, requiring gentamicin:[7] Common regimen is 80 mg 12-hourly IV for 7 days = 14 doses of 80 mg/case **Estimated need: 5% of cases = 50 cases = 700 doses of 80 mg for IV use (each dose = 1 vial of 2 ml for reconstitution)**	Not absorbed from the gut; given by injection for systemic infections Gentamicin is the aminoglycoside of choice and is used widely for the treatment of serious infections Broad-spectrum but inactive against anaerobes When used for 'blind' treatment of undiagnosed serious infection (sepsis) it is usually given in combination with a penicillin or metronidazol or both **For neonatal sepsis** use ampicillin IV (covers *Listeria*) or penicillin IV plus gentamycin **Neonatal dose**: 25 mg/kg ampicillin or penicillin and gentamycin (age up to 2 weeks: 3 mg/kg 12-hourly; age 2 weeks to 12 years: 2 mg/kg 8-hourly)
Chloramphenicol Preferable to use another antibiotic if available Chloramphenicol is a powerful broad-spectrum antibiotic but it should be reserved for life-threatening infections (if no other antibiotic available) and for typhoid fever	Powder in vials of 1 g/vial (would be better if 500 mg/vial) for reconstitution for IV use	Common regimen is 50 mg/kg for average of 70 kg postnatal woman = 3.5g/day in four divided doses; i.e. about 800 mg 6-hourly for maximum 7 days = 4 vials of 1 g/day = 28 vials/case **Estimated need: 5% of cases = 50 cases = 1400 vials containing 1 g for reconstitution for IV use**	IV use in cases of sepsis (postnatal) often in combination with other antibiotics, also for typhoid fever and meningitis Oral use not generally encouraged If needed, ensure cautious use of chloramphenicol in third trimester ('grey' baby syndrome) and during breastfeeding, as may cause bone-marrow toxicity in infant. During breastfeeding, concentration in milk usually insufficient to cause 'grey' syndrome in baby

Drug[1]	Dosage	Estimated amounts needed/1000 deliveries[2]	Notes
Metronidazole	Used IV, oral and per rectum: IV for sepsis in 100 ml bags at 5 mg/ml (this is heavy, therefore may need to replace with rectal dose of 500 mg) Oral given as 800 mg stat then 400 mg or 500 mg 8-hourly Oral can be given as 1 g or 2 g stat Rectal given 1 g stat for prophylaxis at caesarean section and/or as start of treatment for sepsis	In view of various doses but given that this is a very important and useful antibiotic and also used antenatally estimate need at: (assume overall need in 15% of cases)[8] 15 % rectal doses of 1 g stat then 500 mg 8-hourly for 7 days = 22 doses of 500 mg for rectal use/case for 150 cases = **3300 rectal suppositories of 500 mg** 15% oral use – 400 mg capsules most common, therefore estimate 800 mg stat then 400 mg 8-hourly for 7 days = 22 doses of 400 mg capsules/case for 150 cases = **3300 capsules of 400 mg for oral use**	This is a very important and useful antibiotic for sepsis, prophylaxis at caesarean section and also used antenatally
Nitrofurantoin	Tablets of 100 mg for oral use	Use as 100 mg 12-hourly for 7 days = 14 doses of 100 mg/case **Estimated need: 10% urinary tract infection = 100 cases = 1400 tablets of 100 mg for oral use**	Use antenatally for treatment of urinary tract infections
Cloxacillin (e.g. flucloxacillin)	Capsules of 500 mg for oral use For IV use: powder for reconstitution 500 mg/vial	Oral use: 500 mg 6-hourly for 7 days = 28 capsules/case **Estimated need: 5% cases = 50 cases = 1400 capsules of 500 mg for oral use** Common regimen: IV use: 500 mg 6-hourly for 7 days = 28 doses of 500 mg for IV use = **1400 vials of 500 mg for reconstitution for IV use**	Use postnatally, mainly orally for breast abscess, postoperative cellulites/abscess; some cases of sepsis (staphylococcal) may need IV treatment In neonates, sometimes used for umbilical sepsis or staphylococcal skin infection

Drug[1]	Dosage	Estimated amounts needed/1000 deliveries[2]	Notes
3. Antiretrovirals[9]			
Nevirapine	Mother: tablets 200 mg Neonate: oral suspension 50 mg/5 ml	Basic regimen for prevention of mother-to-child transmission: single 200 mg oral tablet at time of labour for mother and for neonate 2 mg/kg as single dose in first 72 hours (average baby 3.5 kg = 7 mg = < 1 ml/case) **Estimated need: for incidence of HIV 25%:[10] 250 doses of 200 mg oral nevirapine for mothers and 25 vials of 50 mg for neonate**	This regimen only addresses prevention of mother-to-child transmission, not treatment of HIV positive women in pregnancy Consideration will need to be given to country where drugs used to adapt regimen Consideration needed to include drugs for treatment HIV positive mother and neonate
HAART (highly active antiretroviral therapy)			Not included in this list at present
4. Antenatal and postnatal care			
Antimalarials:[11,12] Note NATIONAL GUIDELINES to be followed – i.e. exact drug requirement and regime will depend on geographic location.	Chloroquine tablets (100 mg or 150 mg) **OR** Mefloquine tablets 250 mg **OR** Sulphadoxine pyrimethamine (tablets of 500 mg sulphadoxine and 25 mg pyrimethamine) **AND** Proguanil 100 mg tablets	**Estimated need: Chloroquine prophylaxis** = 300 mg/ week for 1000 women, including postnatal period = 46 weeks = **138,000 tablets of 100 mg or 92,000 tablets of 150 mg** **OR** **Mefloquine prophylaxis** = 250 mg/week = 46 weeks = **46,000 tablets** **OR** **Sulphadoxine pyrimethamine**: 2 tablets twice during pregnancy and once postnatally = 6 tablets/case = **6000 tablets** **AND** **Proguanil** given 1 tablet daily for tropical splenomegaly syndrome:[13] estimate 1% prevalence, 300 days/case: need **3000 tablets**	Choroquine: preferred where *Plasmodium falciparum* sensitive Mefloquine: used in areas with high risk or multiple drug resistance Proguanil used in areas with low risk, sometimes together with chloroquine and used in 'big spleen disease' Sulphadoxine pyramethamine: two or three presumptive treatment doses given during antenatal period where chloroquine resistance is noted or as the preferred national regimen in some countries **Note**: new regimens are continuously being developed In HIV-positive women, prophylaxis for malaria may be adapted

Drug[1]	Dosage	Estimated amounts needed/1000 deliveries[2]	Notes
Nifedipine[22]	Sustained-release tablets of 10 mg OR nifedipine 5 mg tablets	5–10 mg given orally in pre-eclampsia, may need to repeat Then 20–100 mg daily in two divided doses; assume for 30 days maximum **For estimated 5 cases: estimated need: 250 doses of 5 mg/case or 125 doses of 10 mg = 1250 tablets of 5 mg OR 625 tablets of 10 mg**	
Methyl dopa[23]	250 mg tablets	Dose 2–3 tablets daily, on average, up to a maximum of 4 g/day **Estimate 5% cases**[24] **= 50 cases 2 weeks treatment each = 42 tablets/case = 2100 tablets of 250 mg**	Centrally acting antihypertensive May be used for the management of hypertension in pregnancy Adverse effects are minimised if dose less than 1 g/day
Quinine	Tablets of 300 mg (quinine sulfate preferred, as it contains more quinine than bisulphate) IV Quinine dihydrochloride 300 mg/ml = 2-ml ampoule (solution for dilution for infusion)	**Oral** 600 mg 8-hourly for up to 10 days = 60 tablets of 300 mg/case 5% cases= 50 cases **Estimated need: 3000 tablets quinine 600 mg for oral use** **IV dosage:** 20 mg/kg initially (estimate 1200 mg) then 10 mg/kg 8-hourly (estimate 600 mg) for 48 hours then usually switch to oral = approximately 8 ampoules of 600 mg/case **For 50 cases estimate 400 ampoules of 2 ml (= 600 mg/ampoule) of quinine**	Quinine used for multiple drug-resistant *P. falciparum* malaria

Drug[1]	Dosage	Estimated amounts needed/1000 deliveries[2]	Notes
Sulfadoxine pyrimethamine OR **Mefloquine** [25]	Sulfadoxine pyrimethamine (tablets of 500 mg sulfadoxine and 25 mg pyrimethamine) Mefloquine 250 mg tablets	Estimated need for treatment of malaria: Sulfadoxine pyrimethamine in malaria endemic areas estimated case load 25% = 3 tablets as a single dose = **750 tablets sulfadoxine pyrimethamine (tablets of 500 mg sulfadoxine and 25 mg pyrimethamine) for estimated 250 cases** **OR** Mefloquine up to 1 g as a single dose 250 cases = estimate 4 tablets/case = **1000 tablets 250 mg mefloquine**	

Antiobiotics for sepsis/fever covered under section 2 above

Drug	Dosage	Estimated amounts needed	Notes
Ergometrine/ ergometrine with oxytocin (Syntometrine®, Alliance) [26]	Ergometrine maleate 200 micrograms 1-ml ampoule (WHO formulary) Also available: Syntometrine® = ergometrine 500 micrograms plus 5 units oxytocin Ergometrine maleate 500 micrograms/1-ml ampoule (UK formulary)	Prevention of postpartum haemorrhage (PPH) when oxytocin not available: 200 microgram IM stat PPH: 250–500 micrograms slowly IV Assuming oxytocin is available as reserve for selected cases of PPH not responding to oxytocin, estimate 5% = 50 cases at 400 micrograms/case **Estimated need: 100 ampoules of 1 ml ergometrine maleate for IM or IV use of 200 microgram ergometrine/ampoule or 50 ampoules of 500 microgram ergometrine/ampoule)**	Ergometrine requires transport by 'cold chain' and refrigerated storage

Drug[1]	Dosage	Estimated amounts needed/1000 deliveries[2]	Notes
Oxytocin [27]	Oxytocin 10 units/ml, 1-ml ampoules	For prevention of PPH: active management of third stage 10 units given IM = 1000 ampoules 1 ml (10 units) oxytocin **Plus** Use in protracted PPH: repeat boluses of 5 units as needed Then 40 units IV (in 500 ml IV fluids) over 4–6 hours: estimate 5% cases = 50 cases protracted PPH = 250 ampoules of 1 ml (10 units) **Total estimated need: 1250 ampoules oxytocin of 10 units (1 ml ampoules)**	
Carboprost	Carboprost as trometamol salt (Hemabate®, Pharmacia) 250 micrograms/ml 1-ml ampoule for injection	250 micrograms IM repeated up to total of 8 doses (2 g) for protracted PPH with uterine atony **Estimated need: 1% cases = 10 cases and 4 ampoules each = 40 ampoules carboprost of 1 ml each**	
Paracetamol	Tablets 500 mg	**Estimated need: 25% will need 10 tablets = 2500 tablets of 500 mg paracetamol**	Use as analgesic antenatally and postnatally and with fever, e.g. in sepsis, malaria
Pethidine [28]	Pethidine hydrochloride 50 mg/ml 1-ml ampoules for injection	Obstetric analgesia: 50–100 mg IM injection 3-hourly up to 400 mg/24 hours **Estimated need: 25% cases require pethidine at 100 mg each = 500 vials of 1 ml (50 mg)**	Opioid analgesic Pethidine produces prompt but short-lasting analgesia. It is used for analgesia in labour; however, other opioids such as morphine or diamorphine are often preferred for obstetric pain Pethidine is cheaper than diamorphine Midwives may be licensed to give pethidine but not diamorphine Also used postoperatively, e.g. post-caesarean section

Drug[1]	Dosage	Estimated amounts needed/1000 deliveries[2]	Notes
Prochlorperazine (e.g. Stemetil®, Castlemead)	Prochlorperazine mesilate 12.5 mg/ml for injection	Given as 12.5 mg/deep IM injection with pethidine **Estimated need: 25% cases require prochloperazine (with pethidine) at 12.5 mg each = 500 vials of 1 ml (12.5 mg)**	Prochlorperazine usually given together with pethidine to reduce nausea and vomiting
Diamorphine	Powder for reconsitution diamorphine hydrochloride 5-mg ampoule	5–10 mg every 4 hours **Estimated need: 1% of cases = 20 ampoules of 5 mg**	
Naloxone	Naloxone hydrochloride 400 micrograms/ml 1-ml ampoule	Neonate: reversal of respiratory depression resulting from opioid administration to mother 200 micrograms as a single dose at birth (or 60 micrograms/kg) **Estimated need in 1% – 10 cases = 10 ampoules**	
Lidocaine	Lidocaine hydrochloride injection: different concentrations available; suggest use 1% or 2% ampoules (with epinephrine if possible) 20 ml ampoules or 2 ml ampoules to be mixed with glucose	Estimated use 15% = 150 cases using up to 400 mg lidocaine/case = 40 ml 1% solution or 20 ml 2% solution **Best estimate: 20 ml 2% solution/case = 300 ampoules of 10 ml 2% (or other combination)**	A necessary 'drug' for general and emergency obstetric care For repair episiotomy and vaginal tears Estimates of amount needed/1000 pregnant women will vary significantly with type and content of ampoule available
Bupivacaine (for spinal anaesthesia)	Bupivacaine 0.5% hyperbaric solution 5-ml ampoules	Estimated need for spinal anaesthesia[29] in 7% of cases = 70 per 1000 Approximate need/case is 2.5 ml but if in 5-ml ampoules will not be able to reuse **Best estimate: 70 ampoules of 5-ml 0.5% hyperbaric solution bupivacaine needed**	For spinal anaesthesia **! Note**: Important that **hyperbaric (or 'heavy')** bupivacaine is used

Drug[1]	Dosage	Estimated amounts needed/1000 deliveries[2]	Notes
Ketamine	Ketamine hydrochloride 50 mg/ml 10-ml vial = 500 mg	6.5–13 mg/kg with 10 mg/kg given IM gives 15–25 minutes of surgical anaesthesia **Estimate need: 700 mg/case = 2 vials/case** **5% cases = 50 cases = 100 10-ml vials of 500 mg ketamine**	For short-term surgical anaesthesia 12–25 minutes, mainly manual placenta removal
Corticosteroids: dexamethasone, **betamethasone**	Most common preparations are dexamethasone and betamethasone = 1-ml ampoules of 4 mg/1 ml for injection (but different preparations exist) Dexamethasone (for shock) 24 mg/ml vials (5-ml vials available)	**For lung maturity**: Betamethasone 12 mg IM 2 doses 24 hours apart OR Dexamethasone 6 mg IM 4 doses 12 hours apart **Estimate 5% need = 50 cases** Betamethasone: 6 vials of 4 mg/case is simplest regimen = **300 vials betamethasone of 1 ml (each containing 4mg)** **AND** **For septic shock**: Dexamethasone IV 2–6 mg/kg repeated up to 6 hourly Estimate 250 mg = approx 2 vials (5ml with 24 mg/ml)/dose 4 doses each case = 8 vials/case **Estimated need: 1% incidence = 10 cases = 80 vials of 5 ml dexamethasone (24 mg/ml) for injection**	A single course of antenatal corticosteroids should be considered routine for preterm delivery If gestational age less than 34 weeks, corticosteroids (either betamethasone or dexamethasone) are given to improve fetal lung maturity and chances of neonatal survival There is evidence to suggest that betamethasone is more effective in reducing respiratory distress syndrome than dexamethasone[30] Corticosteroids are also used in septic shock

6. Newborn care

Antibiotics for neonatal sepsis included above under section 2			
Tetracycline (eye ointment)[31]	Tetracycline hydrochloride 1% eye ointment	At birth, 1 application of ointment to each eye **Generic amount**	Used as a topical anti-infective for prophylaxis of opthalmia neonatorum caused by *Neisseria gonorrhoea* and *Chlamydia trachomatis*

Drug[1]	Dosage	Estimated amounts needed/1000 deliveries[2]	Notes
Silver nitrate (eye drops)	Eye drops silver nitrate 1% (alternative is 2.5% povidone iodine)	2 drops to eacheye at birth **Generic amount**	1% silver nitrate used as a topical anti-infective for prophylaxis of gonococcal opthalmia neonatorum (or 2.5% povidone iodine) **Note**: used if tetracycline eye ointment not available
Vitamin K	Phytomenadione (vitamin K_1) (Konakion® MM paediatric, Roche) 10 mg/ml in 0.2-ml ampoules	0.1 ml IM at or shortly after birth Incidence of multiple pregnancy 5–50/1000 **Estimated need: 1050 doses IM: 1 mg = at 10 mg/ml give 0.1 ml (i.e. need about 525 ampoules of 0.2 ml each of Konakion Paediatric)** For oral administration check relevant preparation	Note: caution needed to avoid dosage errors with Konakion MM paediatric as it is five times stronger than Konakion Neonatal (which has been discontinued) Giving vitamin K at birth is good evidence-based practice. 1 mg may be given by IM and this prevents vitamin K deficiency bleeding in virtually all babies Alternatively, vitamin K may be given by mouth and arrangements must be in place to ensure that the appropriate regimen is followed: 2 doses of colloidal preparation of phytomenadione 2 mg given in the first week For breastfed babies a third dose is given at 1 month (formula feeds generally contain vitamin K)

Neonatal vaccinations[32]

Diphtheria, tetanus and pertussis (DTP)	3 doses at intervals of 4 weeks; first dose at 6 weeks then at 10 weeks and 14 weeks	**Estimated need: at least 1050 doses of each vaccination** (taking into consideration incidence of multiple births)	
BCG			Given at birth in most resource-poor settings
Hepatitis B vaccine			Only given in certain parts of the world where high incidence of hepatitis B (e.g. Asia)
Poliomyelitis	3 doses given orally at 6, 10 and 14 weeks		

References for Appendix 3

The following texts were consulted for formulations of drugs. Wherever possible, doses and formulations are given in the most practical and appropriate format. The proprietary drug is cited where ever possible.

British Medical Association, Royal Pharmaceutical Society of Great Britain. *British National Formulary*. London: BMJ Publishing Group and RPS Publishing; March 2007 [www.bnf.org].

World Health Organization, International Planned Parenthood Federation, John Snow Inc, PATH, Population Services International, United Nations Population Fund, World Bank. *The Interagency List of Essential Medicines for Reproductive Health*. WHO/PSM/PAR 2006.1; WHO/RHR/2006.1. Geneva: WHO; 2006 [www.who.int/reproductive-health/publications/essential_medicines/index.html].

World Health Organization. *WHO Model Formulary*. 2nd ed. Geneva: WHO; 2004 [http://mednet3.who.int/EMLib/wmf.aspx].

For estimated incidence of disease and complications, standard obstetric textbooks were consulted and reference was made to the following publication:

Johns B, Sigurbjornsdottir K, Fogstad H, Zupan J, Mathai M, Edejer TTT. Estimated global resources needed to attain universal coverage of maternal and newborn health services. *Bull World Health Organ* 2007;85(4):1–8.

Other useful references include:

Newton O, English M. Newborn resuscitation: defining best practice for low-income settings. Trans R Soc Trop Med Hyg 2006;100:899–908.

Note: The estimates used in the table above are based on incidence of complications in the population as a whole. Where drugs are used in a secondary or tertiary hospital or in a fully functioning BEOC or CEOC, the incidence of complications/1000 women delivering in the facility may be higher and estimated need will have to be adjusted accordingly.

Notes

1   In general, those drugs considered to be part of a minimum essential package are given in bold (dark) print – those not in bold can be considered useful additional drugs to have available.

2   To estimate drug need, the overall estimated incidence of life-threatening complications occurring during pregnancy or childbirth has been estimated in line with UN/WHO estimates wherever possible (reference: B Johns *et al.*, 2007). In addition, the estimated needs are based on the expected rate of life-threatening complications occurring in pregnancy or during childbirth in 15% of pregnant women (population-based, i.e. 15% of women estimated to be pregnant in the population). For facilities providing, for example, comprehensive emergency (or essential) obstetric care (CEOC), the percentage of women who deliver at the facility (hospital-based population) and who are admitted with life-threatening complications may be higher than 15% and,

similarly, a facility providing basic emergency (or essential) obstetric care (BEOC) may have a lower percentage of complications. Thus, for CEOC facilities, amounts of drugs needed may be higher than given in the table and for BEOC facilities it may be lower.

3   Up to 15/1000 presumptive neonatal sepsis care and 42/1000 neonatal sepsis management estimated = 57/1000; that is, around 5% (ref. Johns *et al.*, 2007)

4   Interagency List of Essential Medicines for Reproductive Health.

5   5% incidence of syphilis is a relatively high estimate; lower figures are given by the Global Burden of Disease Survey (Harvard University Press, 1996) at 0.04–2.3/1000). Incidences will vary strongly by region.

6   Any cephalosporin will be suitable.

7   Puerperal sepsis estimated to occur in 80/1000 cases overall (ref. Johns *et al.*, 2007) but will vary regionally and will also depend on incidence of HIV. Not all cases of sepsis will require cephalosporin treatment.

8   This includes prophylaxis at caesarean section (5% population-based need, WHO/UN), management of sepsis (estimated 8%), treatment of bacterial vaginosis or *Trichomonas vaginalis* (estimated 6%) (ref. Johns *et al.*, 2007).

9   Type of drug and regimen will vary with country and this will need to be taken into account. Presented here are only antiretrovirals for prevention of mother-to-child transmission. We are conscious of the fact the need for treatment drugs for mothers is not addressed in this table.

10   Incidence to be adjusted according to national estimates of prevalence.

11   In malaria endemic countries, antenatal prophylaxis (presumptive treatment) is mandatory. Different regimens are used in different countries according to sensitivity pattern.

12   In malaria endemic areas, antimalarials also needed to treat malaria (dosage given under drugs group 5 below).

13   The prevalence of tropical splenomegaly syndrome is closely linked to endemicity of malaria. Most published figures are from West Africa, where estimates of prevalence vary between 0.5 and 2%.

14   In many cases, iron and folic acid will be needed to treat anaemia. This requires a higher dosage; e.g. iron tablets three times a day. The estimated need above takes this into consideration – it us unlikely that all 1000 women will take full 7 days and 46 weeks of iron/folic acid prophylaxis during pregnancy. Therefore, the estimate is based on 32 weeks/woman in this table.

15   Estimated drug need for treatment of oral candidosis, especially, will be related to prevalence of HIV and AIDS in the population.

16   These tetanus toxoid doses assume that none of the women would have been immunised earlier. If antenatal attendance is high, women may need only an extra two doses each.

17   Note that, if tertiary/secondary referral hospital and/or CEOC /BEOC centre, incidence of (pre-)eclampsia in hospital population may be higher; in such cases may be prudent to double the estimated needs of drugs and or adjust according to incidence in hospital population.

18   This is likely to be an overestimate. If magnesium sulphate is used according to guidelines it is unlikely that calcium gluconate will be needed.

19   Diazepam is to be used only if magnesium sulphate is not available and/or if repeat dose of magnesium sulphate does not work.

20 This is likely to be an overestimate. If magnesium sulphate is used according to guidelines it is unlikely that diazepam will be needed.

21 There is evidence to suggest that, when a maintenance dose is needed, labetalol may be the preferred drug.

22 Decision to revert to nifedipine is to be made at senior level, as this drug can interact with magnesium sulphate.

23 Used antenatally in the case of hypertension not requiring immediate delivery.

24 Based on estimates given in paper by Johns et al., 2007.

25 Note also antimalarial drugs under antenatal/postnatal care. It is important to note that different regions or countries will require different drugs depending on malaria epidemiology; drug regimens do change with emergence of new resistance patterns and new drugs.

26 Oxytocin is generally advised for emergency situations, as it is more stable than ergometrine.

27 In the context of active management of the third stage of labour, skilled attendants should offer oxytocin for prevention of PPH in preference to oral misoprostol. Strong recommendation, high quality evidence: WHO Recommendations for the Prevention of Postpartum Haemorrhage 2007 [http://whqlibdoc.who.int/hq/2007/WHO_MPS_07.06_eng.pdf] for full report.

28   Naloxone is no longer recommended as first line of action for respiratory depression in the neonate as result of opioid administration to the mother; for the neonate, ventilation/ambu bag preferred.

29 Estimated need for caesarean section for obstructed labour = 45/1000, caesarean section for prolonged labour 7/1000, caesarean section for antepartum haemorrhage 1.1/1000, caesarean section for fetal distress 5.6/1000, hysterectomy or uterine repair 2/1000, manual removal of placenta 10/1000. Total estimated need for spinal anaesthesia based on these figures is thus about 70/1000 or in 7% of women (ref. Johns *et al.*, 2007).

30 Roberts D, Dalziel S. Antenatal corticosteroids for accelerating fetal lung maturity for women at risk of preterm birth. *Cochrane Database Syst Rev* 2006 Jul 19;(3):CD004454.

31 According to WHO formulary, this is the preferred prophylaxis for opthalmia neonatorum. Silver nitrate drops or povidone iodine drops maybe used instead if tetracycline is not available. However, in many countries, neither tetracycline eye ointment nor silver nitrate drops are no longer routinely used.

32 This includes all vaccinations which should be given in first 4–6 weeks of life. These are generally the remit of immunisation programmes.

Background reading

American Academy of Family Physicians. Advanced Life System Support in Obstetrics (ALSO) [www.aafp.org/x692.xml].

Cochrane Collaboration. *Cochrane Database of Systematic Reviews* [www.cochrane.org/reviews/en/topics/87.html].

Cox C, Grady K, Howell C, editors. *Managing Obstetric Emergencies and Trauma: The MOET Course Manual*. 2nd ed. London: RCOG Press; 2006.

Enkin M, Keirse MJ, Renfrew M, Neilson J. *A Guide to Effective Care in Pregnancy and Childbirth*. 3rd ed. Oxford: Oxford University Press; 2000.

Johnson R, Taylor W. *Skills for Midwifery Practice*. Edinburgh: Churchill Livingstone; 2000.

Klein S. *A Book for Midwives. A Manual for Traditional Birth Attendants and Community Midwives*. California: Hesperian Foundation; 2000.

World Health Organization. *Making Pregnancy Safer: The Critical Role of the Skilled Attendant. A joint statement by WHO, ICM and FIGO*. Geneva: WHO; 2004 [www.who.int/making_pregnancy_safer/en].

World Health Organization. *Managing Complications in Pregnancy and Childbirth*. Integrated Management of Pregnancy and Childbirth. Geneva: WHO; 2003.

World Health Organization. *Managing Newborn Problems: A Guide for Doctors, Nurses and Midwives*. Integrated Management of Pregnancy and Childbirth. Geneva: WHO; 2003 [www.who.int/reproductive-health/publications/mnp/mnp.pdf].

World Health Organization. *Pregnancy, Childbirth, Postpartum and Newborn Care: A Guide for Essential Practice. Integrated Management of Pregnancy and Childbirth*. Geneva: WHO; 2003.

World Health Organization. *Preventing Prolonged Labour: A Practical Guide. The Partograph Part II. User's Guide*. Geneva: WHO; 1994 [www.who.int/reproductive-health/publications/partograph].

World Health Organization. The WHO Reproductive Health Library [www.rhlibrary.com].

Index